LIVING WITH HIGH BLOOD PRESSURE

DR TOM SMITH has been writing full time since 1977, after spending six years in general practice and seven years in medical research. He writes regularly for medical journals and magazines and has a weekly column in the Scottish *Sunday Mail* and the *Bradford Telegraph and Argus*. He is also the author of *Heart Attacks – Prevent and Survive*, *Coping with Strokes*, and *Coping with Bronchitis and Emphysema* (all Sheldon Press). He is married with two children.

KT-195-315

Overcoming Common Problems Series

For a full list of titles please contact
Sheldon Press, Marylebone Road, London NW1 4DU

Overcoming Common Problems Series

Fight Your Phobia and Win
DAVID LEWIS

Getting Along with People
DIANNE DOUBTFIRE

Getting Married
JOANNA MOORHEAD

Getting the Best for your Bad Back
DR ANTHONY CAMPBELL

Goodbye Backache
DR DAVID IMRIE WITH COLLEEN
DIMSON

Heart Attacks – Prevent and Survive
DR TOM SMITH

Helping Children Cope with Divorce
ROSEMARY WELLS

Helping Children Cope with Grief
ROSEMARY WELLS

Helping Children Cope with Stress
URSULA MARKHAM

Hold Your Head Up High
DR PAUL HAUCK

How to Be Your Own Best Friend
DR PAUL HAUCK

How to Cope with Splitting Up
VERA PEIFFER

How to Cope with Stress
DR PETER TYRER

How to Cope with Tinnitus and Hearing Loss
DR ROBERT YOUNGSON

How to Do What You Want to Do
DR PAUL HAUCK

How to Improve Your Confidence
DR KENNETH HAMBLY

How to Interview and Be Interviewed
MICHELE BROWN AND GYLES
BRANDRETH

How to Love and be Loved
DR PAUL HAUCK

How to Negotiate Successfully
PATRICK FORSYTH

How to Pass Your Driving Test
DONALD RIDLAND

How to Solve Your Problems
BRENDA ROGERS

How to Spot Your Child's Potential
CECILE DROUIN AND ALAIN DUBOS

How to Stand Up for Yourself
DR PAUL HAUCK

How to Start a Conversation and Make Friends
DON GABOR

How to Stop Worrying
DR FRANK TALLIS

How to Survive Your Teenagers
SHELIA DAINOW

How to Untangle Your Emotional Knots
DR WINDY DRYDEN AND JACK
GORDON

Hysterectomy
SUZIE HAYMAN

Is HRT Right for You?
DR ANNE MACGREGOR

The Incredible Sulk
DR WINDY DRYDEN

The Irritable Bowel Diet Book
ROSEMARY NICOL

The Irritable Bowel Stress Book
ROSEMARY NICOL

Jealousy
DR PAUL HAUCK

Learning from Experience
A woman's guide to getting
older without panic
PATRICIA O'BRIEN

Learning to Live with Multiple Sclerosis
DR ROBERT POVEY, ROBIN DOWIE
AND GILLIAN PRETT

Living Through Personal Crisis
ANN KAISER STEARNS

Living with Grief
DR TONY LAKE

Overcoming Common Problems Series

Living with High Blood Pressure
DR TOM SMITH

Loneliness
DR TONY LAKE

Making Marriage Work
DR PAUL HAUCK

Making the Most of Loving
GILL COX AND SHEILA DAINOW

Making the Most of Yourself
GILL COX AND SHEILA DAINOW

Making Time Work for You
An inner guide to time management
MAREK GITLIN

Managing Two Careers
PATRICIA O'BRIEN

Meeting People is Fun
DR PHYLLIS SHAW

Menopause
RAEWYN MACKENZIE

The Nervous Person's Companion
DR KENNETH HAMBLY

Overcoming Fears and Phobias
DR TONY WHITEHEAD

Overcoming Shyness
A woman's guide
DIANNE DOUBTFIRE

Overcoming Stress
DR VERNON COLEMAN

Overcoming Tension
DR KENNETH HAMBLY

Overcoming Your Nerves
DR TONY LAKE

The Parkinson's Disease Handbook
DR RICHARD GODWIN-AUSTEN

Say When!
Everything a woman needs to know about
alcohol and drinking problems
ROSEMARY KENT

Self-defence for Everyday
Practical safety for women and men
PADDY O'BRIEN

Slay Your Own Dragons
How women can overcome
self-sabotage in love and work
NANCY GOOD

Sleep Like a Dream – The Drug-Free Way
ROSEMARY NICOL

A Special Child in the Family
Living with your sick or disabled child
DIANA KIMPTON

Stop Smoking
BEN WICKS

Talking About Anorexia
How to cope with life without starving
MAROUSHKA MONRO

Talking About Miscarriage
SARAH MURPHY

Think Your Way to Happiness
DR WINDY DRYDEN AND JACK
GORDON

Trying to Have a Baby?
Overcoming infertility and child loss
MAGGIE JONES

**Understanding Obsessions and
Compulsions**
A self-help manual
DR FRANK TALLIS

Understanding Your Personality
Myers-Briggs and More
PATRICIA HEDGES

Vasectomy and Sterilization
Making the right decision
SUZIE HAYMAN

A Weight Off Your Mind
How to stop worrying about your
body size
SUE DYSON

Why Be Afraid?
DR PAUL HAUCK

You and Your Varicose Veins
DR PATRICIA GILBERT

You Want Me to Do *What*?
A guide to persuasive communication
PATRICK FORSYTH

Overcoming Common Problems

LIVING WITH
HIGH BLOOD PRESSURE

Dr Tom Smith

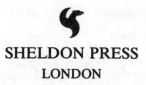

SHELDON PRESS
LONDON

First published in Great Britain in 1985 by
Sheldon Press, SPCK, Marylebone Road, London NW1 4DU

New Edition 1991
Fourth impression 1994

Thanks are due to *The Lancet* and Professor J.D. Swales for
permission to quote from a letter published in *The Lancet* in
August 1984; and to the Williams and Wilkins Co., Baltimore,
for permission to quote from *Clinical Hypertension* by Professor Norman Kaplan (3rd ed., 1982).

British Library Cataloguing in Publication Data

Smith, Tom
     Living with high blood pressure. – (Overcoming common
     problems)
     1. Hypertension – Treatment
     I. Title II. Series
     616.1′3206 RC685.H8

ISBN 0 85969 633 2

Typeset by Inforum Typesetting
Printed in England by Clays Ltd, St Ives plc

Contents

Introduction

If you have high blood pressure, or someone close to you has it, then this book is for you. It explains what blood pressure is, why it needs to be treated, how your doctor keeps it under control and, most important of all, what you can do to help yourself. Like many longstanding bodily upsets – diabetes is another good example – how you cope with high blood pressure is ultimately up to you, and not to your doctor. Your life-style is as important as the treatment you are prescribed.

The first reaction to the news that you have high blood pressure is usually a mixture of fear and surprise. Fear because you may have heard that it carries a risk of heart attacks and strokes. Surprise because you may not feel in any way unwell. For, contrary to popular belief, high blood pressure usually causes no obvious symptoms – not even a headache.

The second reaction is to ask: why me? Have I done something to cause it, and if so, is there anything I can do to reverse the process?

The third is usually: so what? I've been told that I have high blood pressure, but I feel fine – so why should I bother taking treatment which may make me feel worse than I do today? It is a good point, and not easy to answer.

While you are pondering on these questions, you may like to consider another: why do doctors and life insurance companies take rises in blood pressure so seriously? Even a modest rise from normal is likely to 'load' your life insurance premiums, and make your doctor ask you to return every month for a check up.

This book answers all of these questions – and more. It also takes five typical people – and one not so typical person – with high blood pressure, and follows through their case histories from the beginning. If you have high blood pressure, you will almost certainly recognize similarities between yourself and one of them, and will get an insight into the various routine tests and types of treatment. You may, in fact, prefer to go straight to Chapter 2 and read these case histories before getting to grips with more technical information in the first chapter.

This book as a whole explains what high blood pressure is, what we know about its various causes, what happens when it is neglected, what we ourselves can do about it, and what drug treatments are used. Taking drugs that may have side-effects for a long time for an illness that previously has not made you feel in any way ill is not to everyone's liking, so the benefits and drawbacks of drug treatments are described in detail. An understanding of why your doctor has prescribed a particular treatment, its effects and possible side-effects, is always helpful, and particularly so for high blood pressure.

The most important chapters, however, relate to what you can do for yourself to keep your pressure down to reasonable levels. It may mean a whole new approach to life for you – in diet, in exercise, in how you cope with, or can avoid, the stresses which may push it up. Your ambitions, how you relate with colleagues at work, or with your family, the way you react to everyday events, may all have to be reviewed.

However, the last thing you should do is to feel sorry for yourself. Instead, consider yourself very lucky. You have almost certainly found that you have high blood pressure before you have been damaged by it, and you have been given an opportunity to take stock of your life and your health. Everyone, regardless of the height of their blood pressure, should be doing the same.

1

The Facts about
High Blood Pressure

High blood pressure is so common today that most people have at least heard of it, and all too many have either first-hand experience of it or know someone else who has. But many more, including people who – unknowingly – have the condition, have only the vaguest idea what is meant by 'high' blood pressure, or what it entails. So, in this chapter I explain the condition, along with its known causes, and what are believed to be possible causes.

Defining high blood pressure

Your circulation can be likened to two closed systems of pipes within which the blood is driven by a pump, the heart. Your blood pressure is the force that drives the blood through the larger system, taking the blood round the body, and through the smaller system taking the blood between the heart and the lungs – but under much lower pressure. To understand what is meant by 'high' blood pressure it is helpful first to know what is 'normal', and indeed what is 'low' blood pressure.

Normal blood pressure
The blood pressure has two components – the driving force (called the systolic pressure), exerted on the blood by the contraction of the muscle of the heart, and the resistance, or tension (called the diastolic pressure), in the walls of the smaller blood vessels through which the blood flows, and which drives the blood on as the heart relaxes between beats. The 'blood pressure' is a measure of these two forces. Systolic pressure is always higher than diastolic

pressure, and the blood pressure rises and falls between the two with each heart beat. At the outlet of the heart into the system is the aortic valve which prevents any back flow of blood from the vessels into the heart as it relaxes.

The height of blood pressure is measured in millimetres of mercury (mm Hg) – and in adults it will normally be around 130 to 140 systolic, and 70 to 90 diastolic. Blood pressure is usually written as a ratio of the two pressures so that, for example, one of 135/80 simply means that the systolic pressure is 135 mm Hg and the diastolic is 80 mm Hg. In children, blood pressure is slightly slower – usually around 90/60.

Both pressures are measures on an instrument called a sphygmomanometer, which entails wrapping a cuff round the arm, and using a stethoscope to listen to changes in the sounds of the pulse in the arm as the pressure is lowered down the marked scale. More detailed information about the sphygmomanometer and its use is given in the Appendix.

Normally, your blood pressure remains steady through quite a narrow range. During exercise or under stress, it goes up, but when you lie back and relax it should fall again. Only when blood pressure remains well above normal without the stimulus of exercise or stress is a person considered to have high blood pressure, or 'hypertension'.

Low blood pressure
A few people have low blood pressure – that is, their normal blood pressure readings are consistently below 100/60. This rarely causes problems, except for the occasional feeling of faintness and tiredness. Faints occur when there is a sudden drop in blood pressure from the normal to levels which do not sustain the blood supply to the brain, but as soon as the person is horizontal, the flow to the brain returns, and so does consciousness. The fainting attacks are harmless, unless an injury is sustained during the fall.

Most people with low blood pressure, however, have no

symptoms, and only find out about it when their pressure is measured at a routine examination. There is no need for treatment, except in the rare case when fainting attacks are disrupting enjoyment of life.

High blood pressure
One of two changes (or both) in the mechanics of normal blood pressure, could lead to hypertension:

● the first is the heart beating with too much force – which would raise the systolic reading.

● the second is when the small blood vessels become abnormally narrow, raising the resistance to flow of blood through them, and increasing the diastolic pressure.

In high blood pressure, both pressures are usually raised, although only the systolic pressure may be raised in the elderly. On the whole, a rise in the diastolic pressure is more serious than a systolic pressure rise. There is a tendency to classify 'hypertensives' (people with hypertension) as 'mildly affected' if their diastolic pressure is between 95 and 104 mm Hg, as 'moderate' hypertensives if it is between 105 and 114 mm Hg, and as 'severe' cases if it is 115 mm Hg or more.

The vast majority of hypertensives are in the mild category, and the aim is to bring the others, as far as possible, at least down to this level. Initially, the main way of doing this is by drugs with one of two actions – some reduce the force of the heart beat, lowering the systolic pressure; others open up the narrowed small blood vessels to lower the diastolic pressure. Some drugs do both, and some seem to act on the control centres in the brain and nervous system, re-setting the pressure in the system at a lower level. Their actions are explained in detail in Chapter 7.

Causes of high blood pressure

The height of the blood pressure depends on several related nervous and chemical mechanisms, any one of which may be out of balance. The changes that lead to a blood pressure problem in any individual, however, are difficult to detect, and the experts still argue about them. All agree, however, on one thing – that for most hypertensives, the exact chemical or nervous change that has produced the high pressure is irrelevant to the treatment. A patient's body chemistry and nervous system can seem quite normal, but his or her blood pressure is just set at 'high', in which case the diagnosis is 'essential' hypertension.

In a minority – about one in twenty – of people with hypertension, the disease has started with obvious kidney trouble. Knowing how the kidney works is vital to an understanding of high blood pressure, as it may hold the clue even to the cases described as 'essential' although, to date, that clue has not been recognized.

The kidneys' role

The kidneys are a powerful influence on the height of the blood pressure. When the blood pressure falls, as it does during sleep, for instance, they secrete into the bloodstream a chemical called renin, which sets off a chain of chemical reactions in the blood. The final link in this chain is the production of another chemical called angiotensin, which causes the small blood vessels to narrow – producing a sharp rise in the diastolic pressure. The renin system keeps the blood pressure at the correct level. However, an excessive activity of this chemical mechanism is sometimes important in raising the blood pressure. This has led to the introduction of drugs called angiotensin blockers which cut across the chain and successfully treat hypertension. These drugs are described in more detail in Chapter 7.

Kidneys damaged by repeated infections, whether these

were obvious, like Gail's or quite 'silent' like Louise's (see case histories in Chapter 2), often produce excess amounts of renin, which may explain the hypertension. Excess renin production by a kidney starved of oxygen is also the explanation for high blood pressure due to narrowing of the blood vessel feeding it with oxygen and nutrients.

The kidneys also control the volume of salt and water in the body, and in the bloodstream. This is closely linked with blood pressure changes. The more salt is retained in the body, the more water is retained with it, increasing the total volume of body fluids and the pressure in the circulation. Part of this also depends on the renin system. Renin from the kidneys reaches the adrenal glands, which lie across the upper surface of the kidneys. The adrenals respond by releasing another chemical, aldosterone, which causes the kidneys to retain salt and water and raises the blood pressure. This action can be stopped or prevented by drugs (aldosterone antagonists) which block the production of aldosterone by the adrenal glands. For more information on these drugs, see Chapter 7.

Salt retention
In recent years, doctors at Charing Cross Hospital, London, have suggested that people with high blood pressure have a fundamental defect in their bodies' ability to get rid of salt, and therefore water. This leads to the high blood pressure, which can be reduced by putting them on very low salt diets (see also Chapter 4). But the theory is still very controversial since the actual defect responsible has not yet been fully identified. Some doctors deny that it exists.

Chemical imbalance
A very small number of cases of high blood pressure are causes by an enlargement and overactivity of one of the adrenal glands. Called a phaeochromocytoma – the name describes the multicoloured appearance of the gland under

a microscope – it produces excessive amounts of two chemicals called adrenaline and noradrenaline, which together cause the heart to pump harder and the blood vessels to constrict. The result is a massive increase in blood pressure that causes sufferers to have bouts of flushing, palpitations, sweating and headaches. The diagnosis is made from urine tests that reveal traces of the offending chemicals. This type of hypertension needs special treatment, either surgery or medicines, to neutralize the effects of the adrenal gland secretions.

However, most experts in hypertension think that the disease may have several causes, and that no single, overall, cause will be found for it. This explains why a variety of treatments have been devised for hypertension (these are described in Chapter 7). It also explains why self-help plays an important part in its control.

Other considerations

Knowing about the chemical changes in hypertension is all very well, you may say, but how do we acquire such defects in the first place? Are they inherited, or picked up after birth, because of a wrong diet, or caused by some environmental factor, such as a germ or chemical in food?

Answering these questions is not easy. Studies of the blood pressure in relatives of people with hypertension have not led to a clear definition of how it is passed on from one generation to another, if indeed it is.

Heredity
Most cases of hypertension, it seems, are simply extensions of the normal variation in a bodily measurement. Just as a man of 6 ft 4 in would be considered very tall, a person with a blood pressure of 155/95 is at the high end of the statistics for blood pressure. The difference between them is that the extra height does no harm, but the high blood pressure is less innocent.

The tendency to have high blood pressure, like the tendency to be tall, *does* run in families but, as with height, there are many variations within a family. Nevertheless, the more closely you are related to someone with high blood pressure, the more likely you are to have it, too. If your identical twin has hypertension, you are much more likely to have it yourself than would be the case if your twin was non-identical, or if your non-twin brother or sister has it. Also, the children of parents with high blood pressure are more likely to get it than children of parents with normal blood pressure.

Because of the tendency to high blood pressure within families, doctors now ask new hypertensives about their family histories – going back one or two generations sometimes to determine the causes of deaths that might have been due to the disease. More important, if you have hypertension, make sure that your children have regular checks of their blood pressure – if a rise in pressure can be caught early, and steps taken quickly, they should be spared the later complications.

You can do nothing about your heredity, but there are harmful influences on your blood pressure that you can avoid, and these are detailed below.

Diet and hypertension

People with high blood pressure often ask questions about their diet. Am I eating the correct foods? Is one particular constituent of my diet (the usual doubts are about red meats) likely to raise my pressure? Could my hypertension be a reaction to a group of foods – such as shellfish – or to food preservatives? Is there any form of restricted diet that would bring down my pressure without the need for drugs?

The fact is that it does not seem to matter *what* you eat, provided that it is in moderation, and not heavily salted. The only real links ever established between diet and high blood pressure are with excessive consumption of salt, and with gluttony.

9

Salt The bad effects of salt were known to the ancient Chinese. Four thousand years ago, a Chinese physician named Huang Ti, wrote that too much salt 'hardens the pulse' – which may have been as near as the ancients got to describing high blood pressure.

The American professor, Lot Page – an apt Christian name considering the subject of his lifetime's research! – has described at least twenty societies in which high blood pressure is unknown. They have only one thing in common – their consumption of salt is tiny. They range from the wholly carnivorous Eskimo and Masai to virtually vegetarian societies in Iran. Societies in which large amounts of salt are consumed, such as the Japanese, and the Kashkai of Southern Iran, have a high incidence of hypertension, and very high death rates from stroke.

Since 1980, hypertension research has again centred on salt, partly in an effort to avoid the need for long-term treatment with drugs, or at least to lower their dose. Trials of low salt diets have had either spectacularly successful or completely negative results, and this conflicting evidence has left the medical profession undecided on the best advice to give. More is written about this in Chapter 4.

Obesity At least as important as the amount of salt you eat is the total amount of food you consume each day. Gluttony, sadly, is the greatest sin for the hypertensive. The more you are overweight, the higher your blood pressure will be. If you are three or four stones overweight, losing the extra poundage could well bring down your blood pressure to normal, too. Success may depend on how you do it. Simply starving yourself is usually no answer – you can't keep it up, and you will binge yourself back to your old weight, or more. You need to change your eating habits (the best way to do this is described in Chapter 4), and start a sensible programme of exercise. Exercise, provided it is the right kind, and planned correctly, will in itself make you fitter, and help to keep your resting blood pressure lower.

Constipation On the subject of diet, a good piece of advice: do not let yourself become constipated. The act of straining down to expel a hard, constipated stool pushes up your blood pressure quickly, sometimes to alarming levels. If you already have a blood problem, this may even put that little too much strain on that artery in the heart or in the brain, precipitating a heart attack or stroke. It is not a coincidence that many people die while trying to open their bowels – King George III is said to have done so. So make sure that your new diet contains plenty of roughage, so that your stools are soft and bulky, and easy to pass. A good high fibre diet is highly recommended, and is described in Chapter 4.

Smoking and alcohol No consideration of eating habits is complete without a mention of smoking and alcohol – although they are rarely thought of as affecting nutrition by those who indulge in them.

Smoking raises the blood pressure only temporarily; the rise is not sustained, and smoking cannot be blamed for the height of the blood pressure in any individual with hypertension. However, smoking does have several directly harmful effects on the heart, and these are described in detail in Chapter 4. When a heart is already under strain from high blood pressure, smoking is a recipe for disaster. So hypertension and smoking, even of only a few cigarettes a day, definitely do not mix.

In contrast, alcohol, in moderation, does not appear to worsen the effects of hypertension. It depends, of course, how you define 'moderation' (see Chapter 4). Suffice it to say here that most people who drink socially, and think they have no alcohol problem, may find a doctor's definition of 'moderation' to be too conservative for their liking.

Drinking more than a moderate amount of alcohol does raise the blood pressure, and can accelerate the effects of the disease. If you have high blood pressure it is vital to be honest with yourself, and review your intake of alcohol in the light of what is written in Chapter 4. If you drink too much – 20 standard drinks a week is the upper limit for continued good health – and decide to stop, you can do so reassured that your high blood pressure will fall, and remain at the lower level for as long as you abstain.

Emotional factors
Though it can be said that emotional stress does raise blood pressure for a short time, the reaction disappears again as the cause of the stress disappears. Even if you are unhappy at work, or have anxieties at home, there is no proof that they in themselves cause sustained high blood pressure. Only if the stress becomes permanent, and there seems no way of overcoming it or avoiding it, will you get hypertension so constant that it becomes a risk. If this describes your own case, then you need to learn to cope properly with your stress, and ways of doing this are described in Chapter 5, which is devoted to the effect that different reactions to stress have on high blood pressure.

Suppressed anger is probably a more destructive emotion with regard to your blood pressure than either anxiety or depression, and the evidence for this is given in Chapter 5. Suppressed anger may well keep pressure high, through the extra adrenaline released by constantly stimulated adrenal glands. But relaxation, self-knowledge and meditation may be useful, and Chapter 5 also describes how you can practise them.

Drugs that cause high blood pressure
It may come as a surprise, but some drugs can cause high blood pressure:

● Severe high blood pressure has been reported as a reaction to a constituent of a capsule sold to suppress the symptoms of the common cold. Although most of the people reporting the reaction appeared to have taken many more capsules than recommended, if you have high blood pressure, it is sensible to consult your doctor about the drugs you may and may not use as home remedies. Drugs to be particularly careful about include those that constrict blood vessels – such as nose decongestants, even in spray form.

● The combined contraceptive pill can raise the blood pressure. Sue's case (described in Chapter 2) is typical. The hormones is this form of the pill may interfere with the renin system, causing salt and water retention in the tissues and circulation. This explains the bloated, swollen feeling that some women experience when they first start taking the pill.

The hormone doses in the newer combined pills are much smaller, so that fewer women react to them with high blood pressure. However, it is still important for any woman to have her pressure checked several times in the first year after starting on any contraceptive pill. Thereafter, a check once every six months is probably sufficient.

● The same hormones are often prescribed for menopausal troubles, but in amounts very much smaller than those in the contraceptive pill, and rarely lead to high blood pressure. Nevertheless, if you contemplate undergoing hormone treatment for the menopause, it is wise to have your blood pressure checked first.

● Mono-amine oxidase inhibitors (called MAOIs), a group of drugs now prescribed relatively rarely, and only to people with severe depression unresponsive to other treatments, are known to cause sudden bouts of very high blood pressure when taken with certain foods. The combination of the MAOI and a constituent of the foods greatly enhances the effect of natural adrenaline in the body – causing both systolic and diastolic pressures to rise very steeply, sometimes dangerously so.

People given MAOIs are usually warned that they must not drink wines or beer, or eat cheeses, pickles,

13

sauces, and yeast extracts. If you are prescribed an MAOI, make sure that your doctor supplies you with a list of the forbidden foods.

From this survey you will appreciate that there is no single cause of high blood pressure. It has many, and often several are combined. Furthermore, even the most exhaustive tests and questioning often fail to pinpoint a curable cause. Only a small minority are fortunate enough to have the disorder removed by surgery, or by correction of a medical complaint. But that does not mean that nothing can be done by you, or for you, to improve your condition.

Some idea of the diversity of blood pressure problems is given in the next chapter, in which are described typical case histories of hypertension and their various treatments. If you have high blood pressure, you are almost certain to recognize yourself in one of the examples.

2

Profiles of High Blood Pressure

High blood pressure can hardly be called a disease, in the sense that it does not normally produce any sign of ill-health – no symptoms that disturb your normal feeling of well being. It is almost always discovered at some form of routine medical examination, perhaps for a life insurance, or at a first visit for family planning advice or pregnancy.

This is why the diagnosis usually comes as a surprise, and is greeted with some disbelief. If that is your experience, you are not alone. Your story probably bears similarities to that of one of the six people described below.

High blood pressure in young adult life

John is a 27-year-old junior executive in a large manufac-turing company, and is working his way up the ladder, with his sights on a good managerial position by the time he is thirty-five. He works hard, plays hard – squash once a week at the local sports complex, and the odd night out with the lads – but he is a devoted family man, with a good home life, happily married and with a son and daughter, both under school age.

His need to accommodate his growing family in a bigger and better house led them to seek a mortgage, and that required an insurance medical. He thought this was just a formality – after all he felt very fit, and had not seen his doctor for more than five years. In fact, he did not even know his doctor, with whom he had registered after his marriage.

This was all to change, and he is now getting to know his doctor very well. For the insurance medical was not just a formality. The letter from the building society did not contain the expected offer of a mortgage at the normal rate, but a polite refusal. He was given no reason, but was advised that a copy of the examining doctor's report would be sent to his own doctor.

Medical tests – and questions
The mortgage refusal upset him, as he was a natural worrier at the best of times, so that his quickly arranged appointment with his doctor did not go well. He learned that the blood pressure reading taken at the insurance medical had been too high for the insurance company to take him on as a good life risk – and the first reading taken by his own doctor confirmed that he had a problem.

John was then asked to rest for five minutes on the examination couch, while his doctor explained something of the nature of high blood pressure, all the time reassuring him, and persuading him to relax. When his pressure was measured a second time, it was somewhat lower, but still too much above the normal to be ignored.

Even this, the doctor explained, did not necessarily mean that he had high blood pressure that needed constant treatment. The high reading might simply be a temporary reaction to some stress in his life, and would disappear over the next few days. It might even only be a reaction to having to attend the insurance medical, a reaction which understandably recurred at the surgery appointment.

So the next stage was to check on the blood pressure several times over the next week or so – and not in the charged atmosphere of the doctor's surgery. The district nurse would call at his home and measure John's blood pressure there, at different times of the day. That would give some idea of the pattern of his blood pressure changes at the place where he would be most at rest, and presumably least anxious.

John's doctor questioned him closely about his past and present life. What illnesses had he had, even as far back as his childhood? Were there any illnesses in his family, especially of his father and mother? Were they related to blood pressure problems, such as heart attacks and strokes? Had he ever had kidney or urine trouble? Did he have to get up in the night to pass water – that is, apart from after an evening out for a beer or two with the boys? Had he noticed any change in his health over the last weeks, months, or years? Was his weight changing, up or down? How much did he smoke and drink?

Were there any marriage problems? Were there any points of conflict at home which he had not mentioned? Was the proposed house move, to a new district, a source of anxiety to him?

The doctor also discussed with John his work and the responsibilities and anxieties it imposed on him. Were they a burden?

All these questions were relevant to the possible causes of his high blood pressure, but he was able to answer no to them all. His doctor then performed a brief physical examination, confirming what the insurance doctor had found – that, apart from his blood pressure, he was a fit man. After giving small samples of blood and urine, John was able to leave. On this first visit he was not given any treatment for his blood pressure.

Further tests
A week and three visits from the nurse later, John was back in the surgery. The news was not what he had hoped for. His pressure was still too high for comfort, and his doctor wished to take matters further. The routine urine and blood tests had shown no evidence of any cause for the rise in blood pressure, such as kidney disease, which was as the doctor had suspected.

It looked now as if John was like most people with high blood pressure – there was no obvious cause for it that could be cured. He had to come to terms with the fact that his circulation was simply set at a higher pressure that normal, and that he might need to have it checked regularly and treated for the rest of his life.

However, his doctor did not wish to start treatment without one further effort to find the cause. Starting a man in his twenties on life-long drug treatment for a condition which just might be curable by other means is a heavy responsibility. In a few cases like John's, the cause of the rise in blood pressure can be found and reversed. Some possible causes are:

- Occasionally, a small non-malignant tumour in an adrenal gland is the culprit, producing a chemical to which the heart and blood vessels react by bursts of very high blood pressure. Its presence can be detected from traces of the chemical found in the urine. Remove the tumour, and the blood pressure becomes normal.

- Another cause could be a kink or narrowing in one of the blood vessels leading to a kidney. The kidney responds to the poor blood supply by producing yet another chemical that leads to a constant rise in press-ure. Presumably it is the kidney's mechanism of trying to improve its blood supply. Surgeons can remove the offending narrowed section of the kidney vessel. The result after the operation – a normal blood pressure.

John's doctor therefore sent him to a specialist in blood pressure problems so that these possibilities, admittedly remote, could be ruled out. It meant a series of X-rays to show the kidney blood supply in detail, and two or three days of urine tests in hospital.

Regular treatment and the right attitude
As expected, the tests were negative. John was sent home to be treated by his own doctor – and to be advised what to do, not just about his blood pressure, but about his whole life-style.

He learned that discovering his high blood pressure at a relatively early age was no bad thing. In the weeks after the first shock of learning that he was not 'normal' – whatever that means – he stopped feeling sorry for himself.

He even came to the conclusion that he had been very lucky. His high blood pressure had been found before it had time to do him any damage, and he had been given the opportunity to review his life thus far and his attitudes to keeping healthy. The accidental discovery of his pressure problems had given him as good a chance as anyone else of reaching a healthy old age.

John put off his hunt for a mortgage and a bigger house for six months, until he had settled into his regular treatment routine. Then he applied afresh to the same building society. At the new medical, his blood pressure was normal and this, together with a favourable report from his own doctor, led to his acceptance as a normal risk for a mortgage. You can read about the treatments for high blood pressure patients, and the ways in which they can help themselves, in Chapters 3 to 7.

High blood pressure in pregnancy

Louise is now twenty-seven, and the proud mother of a very active two-year-old girl. She, like John, had little cause to visit her doctor until she married four years ago. Both she and her husband wanted children, and were delighted when she became pregnant.

She felt very well in the first few weeks – apart from the occasional morning sickness, and the tendency to have to go to the toilet more often than normal – so she looked forward to her first visit to the antenatal clinic.

It came as a shock, therefore, to learn at that visit that all was not well. The pregnancy was perfectly normal, in that the baby was growing exactly as her 'monthly' dates predicted. But her blood pressure, taken as a routine at all antenatal visits in every woman, was too high. She would need special care throughout the pregnancy.

A clue to the cause of her high blood pressure was found in another routine test done at each antenatal visit – her urine examination. A trace of protein in her urine made the doctor suspect that she had an infection. This was confirmed two days later by the results of another urine test. Although Louise had had no pain, and no trouble passing urine, she had a heavy infection in her kidneys and bladder.

Louise needed help, both with her blood pressure, and against that infection. Antibiotics safe to use under medical supervision in pregnancy and which would kill the offending germs, were given, and she was instructed to rest at home, to see if her pressure would fall without further treatment.

It did so, but not far enough. Her infection cleared, but her high blood pressure did not. This worried her doctor, for to continue with pregnancy with a high blood pressure can lead to problems, and the drugs normally used to treat high blood pressure are not necessarily safe for the developing baby. He was keen that she would rest, and that she should have a specialist opinion about the cause and the treatment of her condition. She left her job, and was admitted to hospital for a few days for tests.

Kidney infections and blood pressure
There it was found that she did have longstanding kidney trouble. For years, unknown to her, she had had repeated infections in her kidneys – looking back on her teens, she remembered days when she felt 'off colour', and had stayed off school, but she had never felt unwell enough to visit her doctor. The 'off' days often coincided with her periods, so she assumed they were to blame.

In retrospect, these had probably been attacks of infection in the kidneys, and these in turn were responsible for the process which led to her high blood pressure. (See Chapter 1 for the connection between kidneys and the control of blood pressure.) In the years to come, she would need to have her urine checked regularly, perhaps once a month, for infection.

In the meantime, she needed treatment to keep her

blood pressure in check. If she co-operated with her doctors in both these aims, there was every reason to believe that her kidneys would suffer no further damage, and that she could live a completely normal life. She was started on a blood pressure-lowering drug that was known to be safe for her baby.

Louise's first reaction was of relief that her pregnancy could continue, although she remained a little anxious until, after a week of treatment, she had her pressure taken again. This time, it was normal – and she stopped worrying. Her doctor, too, felt easier, though he took special care of her throughout the pregnancy until the baby was born, about a week early, a healthy seven-pounder, perfect in every way.

Drugs and self-help

Two years later, Louise still takes drugs for her blood pressure. The practice nurse measures her pressure every month when she arrives for her repeat prescription, and she sees her doctor for a quick chat, to discuss any problem. Her urine has not been infected for a year, and she has learned a lot about preventing new infections. For example, she showers, instead of lying in the bath at night. (In a woman, germs from the skin can find their way into the bladder, and from there to the kidney, simply if she sneezes or coughs while in the bath. There is no such danger from a shower.)

She takes no added salt at meals, and puts virtually no salt in her cooking. When her daughter goes down for her afternoon nap, Louise settles down on the bed beside her, and she believes that this has done her the world of good. Only now that she feels so fit does she realize how under par she had been before her high blood pressure was discovered.

Her blood pressure is now under excellent control, and over the last year she has needed smaller and smaller doses of her drugs to keep it at normal levels. Her doctor holds

21

out high hopes for her eventually taking no drugs at all – she has an even chance of doing without them – but he stresses that her change in life-style and her regular blood pressure checks must be lifelong.

High blood pressure and the pill

Sue is thirty-six, and has completed her family. Her three children are all at school, and she was looking forward to returning to work. Before she did so, however, she wanted to change her form of contraception. Previously, between her planned pregnancies she and her husband had relied on barrier methods, first sheaths, then a diaphragm.

Now, the contraceptive pill seemed to be the right choice for her – she saw it as the most effective and the most convenient method, and her doctor agreed that there was nothing in her medical history to prevent her taking it. She had always been well, her pregnancies and deliveries had been uneventful, and without any sign of raised blood pressure.

Sue is also a non-smoker. If she had smoked, her doctor would not have been happy to prescribe the pill for her, for the risk of heart disease rises considerably in women in their later thirties who both smoke and take the pill.

A reaction to the 'combined' pill

Her first visit to the doctor for family planning advice went well. She had a thorough physical check-up, including an internal examination and a smear test, her urine was tested for diabetes and kidney trouble, and her blood pressure taken. Everything was normal. She was given a month's supply of one of the standard 'combined' pills, and asked to return four weeks later.

At the second visit her doctor took longer over checking her blood pressure. Nevertheless, she was given a second pack of pills. At the next visit, her doctor dropped a bombshell. Sue would have to come off the pill, because

22

her blood pressure was rising. It was not yet up to even mildly worrying levels, but the slow rise since she started the pill was enough to convince her doctor that it was her body's response to the combined pill.

Most contraceptive pills are of the 'combined' type – that is, they contain both the female sex hormones, progestogen and oestrogen. When a woman starts on the combined pill, her blood pressure rises just a little, but not enough to make any difference to her health. In one woman in forty, however, this rise continues until the pressure is above normal levels – a trend which, continued for years, might lead to trouble. It is thought to be related to the oestrogen, contained in the combined pill.

The 'progestogen-only' pill

Sue had two choices – to return to her old barrier methods, or to try the 'progestogen-only' pill, which might not have the same effect. The progestogen-only pill has less or no effect on blood pressure, and has been used successfully by women for whom the combined pill is unsuitable. It is not quite as reliable, however, and is prescribed usually as a second choice, or for women in their later childbearing years.

Sue decided to try the progestogen-only pill, and has remained well on it. Her blood pressure is back to normal, but she will have it checked every six months until she stops taking the pill, and whenever she returns to her doctor for any illness or advice. Once you are identified as a potential high blood pressure patient, your doctor is always on the alert for any possible rise. The only way to catch a rise before it starts to do harm is to measure it at every visit, regardless of whether there are symptoms or not.

Sue's blood pressure problem was almost certainly a reaction to the hormone in the pill, and will not occur again. She has discussed it in detail with her doctor, and it has led her, as it did with John and Louise, to take stock of her life. She lives more sensibly – with a better attitude to exercise and food – and is more relaxed. She has lost that feeling that the world is passing her by, and has not rushed back, full time, into the business world. She now realizes that would have added stress. Instead, she has taken a part-time job as an adviser, allowing her some time at home during each day.

High blood pressure and mid-life stress

Of our examples thus far, Bill was the only one to go to his doctor because he felt unwell. He is fifty-five years old, and an area sales manager for a large manufacturing company. He had always worked hard, and now had the responsibility of training and supervising more than twenty young sales representatives. He took his responsibilities seriously, and was in keen competition with the eight other area sales managers.

Bill led his team from the front, working harder than anyone else, and even taking less holidays than his full entitlement. A recent take-over at the top of his company, which threatened to result in many redundancies, forced him to work even harder, and to worry even more than usual.

Troublesome symptoms
Bill started to feel ill. He would get the odd pain in the chest on exercise, though it stopped when he rested. From time to time he had a dizzy spell though this, too, cleared quickly when he sat down. Being the man he was, he kept these symptoms to himself, not even confiding in his wife. It was not until his symptoms interfered with his working day that he finally sought his doctor's advice.

What brought him to his doctor's surgery was not the chest pain or the dizziness, but a headache. It was there when he woke in the morning, and sometimes was coupled with blurred vision. This meant that he found it difficult to drive to his morning appointments with his salesmen. Bill

24

needed these headaches sorted out, so that he could get on with his work. Hence the appointment with his doctor.

Bill's doctor had different priorities. The chest pain suggested to her that Bill's heart might be affected; the dizziness that the circulation to his brain needed attention, and the headache and blurred vision pointed to a neglected high blood pressure. She took his blood pressure, listened to his heart, and arranged for a chest X-ray and electrocardiogram (ECG) reading. The ECG is a tracing of the electrical activity of the heart – from which the doctor can establish how much the high blood pressure has affected it. It is painless and not at all frightening. He was given an appointment for a much longer meeting several days later.

At that appointment she was unhappy, to say the least, about the results of the tests, and with what she heard from Bill about the way he lived. His blood pressure was far too high for safety, the chest X-ray showed that his heart was too large, and his electrocardiogram showed considerable evidence of long-term high blood pressure. It also showed that he was possibly heading for a heart attack if the pressure was not brought down fairly quickly.

Drug treatment and rest

Bill was told, in no uncertain terms, that he had to change. His pressure could be brought down without any difficulty, using drugs, but this was useless unless his whole attitude to life changed. He had to delegate more of his responsibilities at work, take more time off, learn to relax, and stop being so competitive. It would be difficult, but he had to unlearn many of the habits that had made him a successful businessman – and she assured him that, properly organized, he could do so without jeopardizing his job.

To start with, she signed him off work for a fortnight, and arranged to have his pressure checked at home. Also, because his pressure was so high, and the symptoms suggested that he might be heading for a stroke or heart attack, she started him on a drug to lower his pressure without waiting for the results of other tests.

After a week, Bill's blood pressure had fallen considerably, but not yet to normal levels. He was already worrying about the work piling up at the office, despite the reassurances of his colleagues that they were coping well. His doctor added a second drug, and increased the dose of the first one. (It often needs more than one drug – with slightly different actions – to control the pressure at the start of treatment. Most doctors start with one drug, then add another if the first is not completely effective. About half of all blood pressure patients need more than one drug, at least initially – see Chapter 7 for a more detailed description of drug treatments). She reinforced her first message, that his health mattered more than his company's profits, and made a mental note to keep him off work for two more weeks.

A new regime – and good results
At the end of the second week, Bill's pressure had fallen further, and she was happier with him. One good sign was that he felt better about his job. His boss from head office had visited him, and had showed great concern: and the fact that two juniors were needed to fill the gap had given his pride a boost.

A month after that first visit, he was allowed to return to work. He now had an assistant sales manager, to take some of the load from him. His blood pressure was under control, and he no longer had chest pains, dizzy spells or headaches.

His doctor was thinking, even at this early stage, of reducing his drug doses. Bill had followed all her advice – especially on stopping smoking, cutting down on his alcohol consumption, and on his work load. Her only worry was how long his good resolutions would last.

High blood pressure from childhood

Of our cross-section of high blood pressure sufferers, Gail stands out in another important respect. She has never enjoyed good health. Only seventeen-years-old now, she had had kidney problems since she was a toddler. Her first symptom, just before her second birthday, was a convulsion – a terrifying experience for her parents, who thought that she was dying.

In fact, she recovered very quickly, and the doctor was able to reassure her parents that the fit was simply due to the high fever she had at the time. Such febrile convulsions are very common in small children, and the tendency almost always dies out before school age.

What was more important to the doctor at that first illness was the cause of the fever. Gail had no obvious cause for the fever, such as a cold or chest infection, nor did she have signs of more serious illness, such as meningitis – an inflammation of the surface of the brain. A sample of urine, however, revealed why she had the fever. She had a severe infection of the bladder, and probably in the kidneys, too.

Legacy of kidney infections

Antibiotics cleared up the infection, but later X-rays showed that Gail had some kidney damage, much of which must have occurred from previous infections producing no, or the minimum of, symptoms. From then on, Gail was often unwell, and needed treatment for repeated kidney infections.

Fortunately, as the years passed she grew out of her infections and her kidneys healed, but scars still showed on her X-rays. In her late teens, she was outwardly as healthy as anyone else, but the kidney damage, though no longer progressing, and unlikely to shorten her life, had left her a legacy of higher than normal blood pressure.

An early start to lifelong treatment

Her doctors pondered on what to do. Should they treat this disorder, of which Gail was unaware, knowing that the treatment might make her feel worse than she felt at the moment, or should they just wait and watch, for a few more years?

On balance, they decided on treatment, for three reasons.

● They knew Gail to be a responsible, intelligent girl, who could take the news that she might need lifelong treatment with calm acceptance, and would understand and co-operate.

● Gail was going away to college. She would have to know everything about herself and the risks she would be taking if she fell ill. The years ahead would presumably include decisions to be made about birth control and pregnancy, and her blood pressure would have a strong bearing on them.

● The evidence is now very strong that the earlier high blood pressure is brought under good control, the better and longer is the expectation of life. The doctor's aim was to give Gail every chance of reaching a happy and healthy old age, by starting to treat her blood pressure, without delay.

Gail took her talk with her doctor well. She started on a course of treatment that has kept her pressure well within the normal limits, and she is in her first year at college, without any restrictions on her academic and leisure activities. She has taken up fun running, and feels fitter than ever. Her blood-pressure-lowering tablets, which she takes once a day, every morning, in no way spoil her enjoyment of life.   •

Solutions for severe cases

Thanks to the better recognition and treatment of kidney

infections in early childhood, cases like Gail's are much less common than they used to be. Gail herself was luckier than some, whose kidneys eventually fail altogether, either because of the damage due to repeated infections, or from other childhood kidney diseases. Happily the kidney dialysis and transplant programme can now deal with them, and with the blood pressure problems they create, but to discuss such measures is beyond the scope of this book.

High blood pressure at sixty-plus

In her late sixties, Doris decided that she was heavier than she would like to be, and made an appointment with her doctor to ask for a reducing diet. She did not feel particularly unwell, though she did occasionally wake up with a dull headache. Now that she was retired, she was physically less active, and this, combined with her healthy appetite, had contributed to a weight gain of more than two stones over the past three years.

Her doctor found that not only was Doris four stones overweight, but she had a blood pressure well into the 'moderate to severe' range. He set about helping her in three ways.

- She was given advice on how to eat sensibly to lose the surplus weight, stressing that this was not so much a diet, but more an attempt to change her attitudes to food and mealtimes (see also Chapter 4).
- She was advised to become more active physically, starting gradually, with short walks, and progressing slowly to more ambitious exercise. It was explained that becoming fitter would tend to lower her blood pressure.
- She was given a low dose of a blood-pressure-lowering drug, and asked to come back weekly for checks.

The gentle approach
As her weight began to fall, so did Doris's blood pressure.

A month after the first visit, she had lost half a stone, and her pressure was now in the 'mildly hypertensive' category. Her drug dose was reduced, and the advice on diet and exercise was re-emphasized. It took her a year to lose two stones, but this was considered very satisfactory by her doctor, especially as by this time she was off all drugs, feeling well, and eating sensibly. She still sees her doctor once a month for a check of her pressure and her weight.

Doris's case is typical of many women who start to put on weight in middle age, at a time when they are becoming much less active. It is so common that doctors used to accept that blood pressure normally rises with age. It would be more true to say that it rises with 'middle-aged spread'! If men and women keep fit – and keep their figures – through their fifties and sixties, they are more likely to keep their blood pressures within the normal range.

When treating older people with high blood pressure, the priority is to bring down the pressure gently and slowly. A rapid fall, as produced by higher doses of the stronger drugs, may bring down the pressure too low, introducing the risk of a thrombosis – and causing the stroke which the treatment is designed to avoid. Happily, the gentle approach works very well in the over-sixties.

If you have high blood pressure, the stories of John, Louise, Sue, Bill, Gail or Doris may be very familiar to you. Together, they are representative of almost every high blood pressure victim in developed countries. They differ widely in the way they discovered that they had a problem, but the medical attention and advice they received on the self-care they would need to practise for the rest of their lives are very similar. Why their co-operation was vital is made clear in the next chapter.

3

Lowering Your Blood Pressure

Why treat high blood pressure at all? This is a perfectly reasonable question, especially if asked by someone who felt well when it was raised before treatment, and then, once the treatment has started, feels terrible.·

The four arguments *against* treating high blood pressure run roughly as follows:

1 Most people with high blood pressure feel well, or at least do not feel ill, and most modern drug treatments can cause side-effects that make them feel worse, despite their blood pressure being lowered to normal.
2 Some people with very high blood pressure live normally into old age without any problems when, by all the statistics, they should have died years before.
3 It is impossible to prove that using drugs to keep a particular individual's blood pressure normal will prolong that person's life.
4 Treating high blood pressure involves not only taking drugs, but changing almost every aspect of one's life. Is the trouble worthwhile?

The best way to answer these arguments is to show the risks you run if your high blood pressure is left uncontrolled. There are two ways of looking at the evidence; we can see what happens to individuals with hypertension as they age, and we can look at the statistics relating to deaths from hypertension all over the world, including those on which life assurance companies base their premium rates. Such figures are very carefully calculated and must be accurate measures of the extent to which hypertension shortens life.

Nevertheless, as must be the same for many other doctors, my own feelings about the decision to treat or not to treat hypertension are based on my experiences with

31

patients as a student and house physician. It is the people we cared for ourselves who shape our individual approach to the treatment of disease.

When I was a student and then a young doctor in the late 1950s and early 1960s, the drugs for high blood pressure were much less effective, and caused many more, and worse, side-effects than those used today. In our medical wards, there were always patients suffering from the last stages of high blood pressure, many of them still young.

I particularly remember two of them. One was a schoolteacher, aged forty, with a loving family and everything to live for, who died of a heart attack after several strokes. The second was a young woman who developed severe high blood pressure in her first pregnancy, and two years later died of kidney failure.

Today, neither would have died. The schoolteacher would have responded very well to the modern drugs and have a normal life expectancy. The young mother would have had her high blood pressure in pregnancy managed much more efficiently, and her kidney failure would almost certainly have been prevented. Even if the kidney trouble could not have been avoided, the dialysis and transplant option would now be available to her.

Even as recently as two decades ago, hypertension often ended as a condition called 'malignant hypertension', with the sufferer going blind, suffering minor strokes, and eventually dying of kidney failure, because of the damage the disease can cause to the circulation. Once this stage was reached, the expectation of life was less than a year, despite the best available treatment.

Yet many doctors who have qualified since the early 1970s have never seen a full-blown case of malignant hypertension, so great have been the improvements in treatments. For me, this is the best argument for active treatment of all cases of high blood pressure. Now that we can keep at bay the complications of the severe form, we should use every opportunity to do so.

How hypertension harms you

For those who need further convincing, below I outline the possible development of the disease, if it is not treated.

The arteries

The blood vessels take the main brunt of the constantly high pressure, and have to change to cope with it. The walls thicken, presumably to withstand the extra force applied to them. Their inner linings, normally smooth to allow fast flow of the blood inside them, become roughened, so that the diameter of the channel through which the blood has to flow narrows.

In these narrowed, roughened, thickened arteries, the blood flow becomes sluggish. The blood itself becomes stickier as it is pushed by the pressure through the narrowed vessels, and tends to clot much more easily than usual. The scene is set for a thrombosis – a lump of solid, clotted blood, attached to the roughened artery wall. If the clot is large enough, it will stop the flow of blood completely – and if it is in an important branch of a coronary artery, the result will be a heart attack. If it is in the brain, the result will be a stroke.

Occasionally, the high pressure ruptures a weakened artery in the brain so that the blood escapes, in a haemorrhage, into the brain substance. Such a cerebral haemorrhage results in a very severe stroke, always leaving some serious after-effects, such as a paralysis, in survivors, and often it is fatal.

The heart

This too, can be damaged by longstanding untreated high blood pressure. In the beginning, it copes with the strain of maintaining the high pressure by increasing its muscle bulk, enlarging so that it can pump harder. Eventually it cannot enlarge any further without losing its efficiency. The continuing high pressure expands and thins it, so that it becomes like an overblown balloon.

At this stage, the pump starts to fail. The heart can no longer drive the volume of fluid in the circulation around the body, and some of it begins to accumulate in tissues such as those in the legs and the lungs. The main symptoms are breathlessness on the least exertion, and swollen feet and ankles. If the swelling is pressed with a finger, a small pit-like depression is left in the waterlogged flesh.

The kidneys

The other organ most affected by longstanding neglect of high blood pressure is the kidney. In the end, the kidneys of people whose blood pressure did not start with kidney disease can be as badly affected as those with kidney damage from the beginning. Constant hypertension thickens the blood vessels in the kidneys, interfering with the very delicate mechanisms which produce urine.

The result is a vicious spiral, in which the kidney function deteriorates, and the hypertension worsens, producing even more kidney damage. One of the first signs of kidney damage due to high blood pressure is a loss of the ability to concentrate urine, so that it becomes necessary to rise in the middle of every night to empty the bladder.

Vision

A small minority of people with high blood pressure have most bother with their eyes. The fine network of tiny blood vessels which supply the retina (the screen at the back of the eyeball that gives us our sight) can be affected in the same way as the circulation in the brain. The pressure inside them may even make them leak fluid into the eye, causing the eyesight to deteriorate rapidly if the blood pressure is not quickly brought under control.

The case for treatment

From the available statistical evidence, the need to treat moderate and severe hypertension is undeniable, since treatment gives many people extra years of life to enjoy. There is more doubt, however, about the need to treat people with mild hypertension, that is, those whose diastolic pressures (see page 5) are between 95 and 104 mm Hg. Can they safely be left with pressures at this level?

Until recently, the usual answer to this question was a guarded 'yes'. Now, many doctors have changed their minds, and are doing everything they can to bring their patients' blood pressures down to normal. Their change in attitudes stems directly from the results of two large trials of modern drug treatment against 'placebo' (dummy) treatment or a more lax regime, in more than 10,000 mildly hypertensive men and women in Australia and the United States, both of which were reported in 1980.

The Australian trial

Some 3,420 subjects were divided into groups of equal numbers, and either given active drugs to bring their blood pressure down into the normal range, or a placebo tablet without any blood-pressure-lowering activity. Only if the blood pressure rose above the 'mild' limit were patients in the placebo group switched to active treatment.

In the course of five years there were four deaths in the group receiving the active drugs, and thirteen among those given the dummy treatment. Such a big difference could not be attributed to chance, and indeed the smaller death rate was entirely due to a large reduction in the deaths from heart attacks and strokes in the group on active treatment. This group also suffered many fewer non-fatal strokes and heart attacks.

The smaller number of deaths in the actively treated group could be directly related to their fall in blood pressure – the average diastolic pressures in the treated group were consistently between 5 and 7 mm Hg below those given the placebo. These may seem small changes, but they were enough to make a clear difference in outcome.

The American trial

This came to a similar conclusion, though it differed from the Australian trial in that every patient received some form of active treatment. Half of the 7,800 patients were treated intensively by the researchers, with the goal of bringing their diastolic pressures below 90 mm Hg, and half were referred back to their own doctors for the usual medical care.

In the following five years the group receiving the extra care had significantly lower blood pressures, and twenty per cent fewer deaths than those sent back to their own doctors. Most of the extra deaths in the 'usual care' group were due to heart attacks and strokes, presumably directly attributable to their higher blood pressures – only about half of this group had been given blood-pressure-lowering drugs.

Summing up the results

The doctors who conducted both these studies came to the very strong conclusion that mild hypertension should be treated as actively as possible. They made several other points, too, which must be of interest to anyone who is trying to cope with his or her own blood pressure problems.

The first was made by Professor Austin Doyle, of Melbourne. He stressed that the figures showed the importance of treating mild high blood pressure before it caused damage to the heart or circulation. Secondly, most of the patients in the placebo group in the Australian trial had a satisfactory fall in their pressures, which Professor Doyle put down to the better care they were receiving by just being on the trial, and trying to do something about their blood pressure. Personal efforts such as losing weight, cutting down on salt, stopping smoking, a better exercise programme, and more relaxation could all have played their part in producing this satisfactory result, and should not be dismissed.

In fact, the Australian patients whose diastolic blood

pressure fell to between 90 and 100 purely on the placebo combined with a more appropriate life-style fared better than those for whom drugs led to the same blood pressure level. The big difference in illness and deaths between the two groups came when the drugs brought the diastolic pressures below 90. Such a fall was rare on placebo alone.

Dr Herbert Langford, of the University of Mississippi, who reported the American results, made the point that the differences in deaths and illnesses between the American groups could be accounted for largely because those receiving the extra care were known to have stuck more closely to their doctor's instructions and took their drugs more regularly.

The progress in drugs for high blood pressure has not simply been in terms of efficiency. Among all the patients in the Australian and American studies – 10,000 followed for up to five years – not a single death or serious illness could be attributed to a side-effect of a drug. Minor side-effects were reported, but no more than would be expected of long-term treatment with any type of drug, and little more than those reported on the placebo.

Finally, the Americans pointed out that most people with hypertension are in the mild group, and most of the deaths due to hypertension in American are in this group. A fall of twenty per cent in deaths in the first five years was an unexpectedly large improvement, which if spread countrywide would prevent tens of thousands of deaths each year.

The Australians calculated their savings in serious complications of hypertension, such as strokes and heart attacks, as seven, and in deaths as two, per 1000 persons per year. In Australia, with its 12 million people, this would mean 7000 fewer complications and 2000 fewer deaths every year if every mild hypertensive were treated. If these figures were applied to Britain, the number of deaths prevented every year would be 9000.

Since 1982 the American and Australian study results have been confirmed by two huge studies reported in the *Lancet* of 31 March and 7 April 1990.

This team of doctors from the United Kingdom, New Zealand and the United States first looked at the death and disease rates in no fewer than 420,000 adults with a wide range of blood pressures, followed for 6 to 25 years.

The height of the diastolic blood pressures was closely related to the risk of stroke and heart attack. Reducing the usual diastolic blood pressure by 5mm reduced the incidence of stroke by 34% and that of heart attack by 21% A fall of 10mm in the diastolic pressure decreased the stroke rate by 56% and the heart attack rate by 37%. The conclusion was that for 'the large majority of individuals a lower blood pressure should eventually confer a lower risk of vascular disease'.

The second report, written by the same group of doctors, analyzed 14 trials of drug treatment of high blood pressure in 37,000 people treated for 5 years. They showed protection against stroke and heart attacks within two years of starting treatment, strokes being reduced by 42% and heart attacks by 14%. In the longer term, the stroke risk continued to be cut by around 40%, and the risk of heart attacks was reduced by between 20% and 25%. The authors concluded that a risk of stroke was the clearest indication for bringing down high blood pressure.

Getting our priorities right

Convinced, then, that we should always do all we can to bring down high blood pressure, even if mild, into the normal range, how should we go about it?

The first priority, all the experts agree, is not drugs. Everyone with high blood pressure will improve to some extent by changing his or her life-style, and some will improve so much that they will never need drugs. Here is Professor Norman Kaplan, of the University of Texas, Dallas, writing in a medical textbook about how he approaches new patients with hypertension:

Everyone should have their blood pressure taken once a year. If it were taken as it should be – at every contact with the health care system – this could be accomplished for most adults without the need for special screening programmes.

If the blood pressure of a person over the age of 16 averages above 140/90 mm Hg at the first set of readings, it should be retaken within a month. If it remains above 140/90 but below 160/110 mm Hg, the patient should be offered general advice; gradual weight loss if obese, moderate salt restriction, regular exercise, and a reduced intake of alcohol if it exceeds an average of 5 ounces a day.

If other heart and circulation risks such as hyper-cholesterolaemia (abnormally high fat levels in the blood), cigarette smoking, diabetes, or oestrogen use are present, they should be addressed [seen to]. The more the overall risk, the more aggressive should be the attempt to lower the blood pressure. If the diastolic blood pressure remains above 100 after 6 months despite these general measures, drug therapy to lower the pressure should begin.

Non-drug therapy will lower the blood pressure to a safe level in many patients with mild hypertension. Though this may partly reflect a progressive fall in blood pressure over time by the simple process of repeating the measurement; weight reduction and sodium restriction will lower the blood pressure, and regular exercise and relief of stress may help.[1]

The next chapter explains in detail how to follow Professor Kaplan's advice.

[1] From *Clinical Hypertension* (Williams & Wilkins Co., 3rd ed., 1982)

4

Diet, Drink and Smoking

Once that you have been told that you have high blood pressure, what can you do about it? The first priority is to recognize that you have your future in your own hands. Only by re-assessing your life, in every way, and by approaching the problems as a partner with your doctor, understanding the reason for each step, and fully committing yourself to the new patterns, will you give yourself the best chance of a long and healthy future.

This chapter deals with diet, drink and smoking habits. The following ones tackle stress and how to cope with it, and exercise. Look at all these measures as equally important; they are complementary, not alternatives!

At first sight, exhortations to modify your diet and social pleasures may seem rather puritan and killjoy. It is tempting to see such advice as simply the doctor's way to make you suffer while you are treated – but don't succumb to that particular temptation. The following recommendations on diet, drink, smoking, relaxation and exercise are based on reasoned assessments of their effects on high blood pressure, from thousands of patients. Many people who have stuck to them have managed to control their blood pressures without the need for drugs, or with much smaller doses of drugs than they would have needed otherwise.

Apart from the effect the new life-style will have on your blood pressure, you will probably be surprised at how much better you will feel. For the first time in years, perhaps, you will learn how good it is to feel really fit.

Adjusting your diet

Over recent years anyone could be excused for being confused at what doctors have said about the proper way to eat. From 'going to work on an egg' and 'drink a pint of milk a day' – the slogans of the 1960s – we have swung round to a position that eggs contain too much cholesterol, and all dairy products have too much animal fat, to be good for you. Bread and potatoes, foods which people used to be told to avoid, are now considered 'healthy'. Today, everyone is exhorted to stick to 'polyunsaturated' vegetable fats and oils, high fibre diets, and white meats and fish rather than the traditional red meats. Lots of fresh vegetables and fruit, polyunsaturated margarines rather than butter, and avoidance of all refined sugars, are the order of the day.

How do any of these instructions relate to your high blood pressure? The simple answer is that they don't! No single food has ever been proven to be directly related to high blood pressure in people, with the exception, perhaps, of salt. And even the link with salt is doubted by some doctors. This does not mean that you don't have to bother about your diet. On the contrary: it is the *sum* of all that you eat that worsens your blood pressure.

Consequences of overweight

The biggest risk to anyone with high blood pressure is to be overweight, and the more extra weight you carry, the larger your risk. If you are more than a stone overweight, your first task is to lose the excess, and your second is to stay at your new, normal weight, for the rest of your life. We will come to the best way to do this shortly, but first it is helpful to know precisely why being overweight is so bad for people with hypertension.

Your heart pumps blood to every minute part of your body relatively by beating – contracting its muscle mass – roughly seventy times a minute. If you are carrying an extra stone or more of fat, it has to increase its power accordingly, to cope with the extra volume of blood vessels, and it has to keep up this extra output for many years. Here is a simple analogy: if you run a car engine too hard, and persistently carry loads too heavy for its design, for many years, you would expect engine and chassis to wear out sooner. This fairly reflects what happens, over years, to the heart in high blood pressure. Remove that extra load, run the engine more smoothly and economically, and you can almost guarantee a longer life for your car – or your heart.

Life assurance companies know this very well. Their figures, of people with normal blood pressures, show that, on average, the overweight die sooner than people of normal weight for their height – and if you lose the extra poundage, you can put off that risk of premature death. The bonus of extra years of life applies particularly to those with high blood pressure.

The Framingham study – in which the whole population of a town in the United States were studied for many years – has shown that being overweight can even lead to the development of high blood pressure. While following the progress of the Framingham townsfolk over the years, the doctors found that among the overweight adults who when first seen had normal blood pressures, three times as many as expected eventually developed high blood pressure. And for every fifteen per cent of weight loss they then achieved, their blood pressures dropped by ten per cent. This is more than enough to save many lives.

How to assess whether you are overweight

Most people do not need to be told. You know if you are too fat, just by looking at yourself in a mirror. You may have struggled with a too-hearty appetite since you were a child, or have put on weight gradually since your mid-twenties, and had more to eat, and took less exercise. That 'middle-aged spread' has been a slow, but not imperceptible, process and is certainly neither 'natural' nor irreversible.

If you need guidance, however, on just how much overweight you are, tables of desirable weights are printed from time to time in a host of magazines. Unfortunately, they are usually divided into 'frame sizes' of large, medium and small – assessments that are not too easy to make for yourself. And many people deceive themselves that they are 'large-framed', whatever that means, because in that category they can weigh rather more than someone of the same height, but of a 'small' or 'medium' frame.

A more reliable method is to see how thick your skin and fatty tissues are around the tummy. If you pinch a roll of tummy skin between your thumb and forefinger, and it is over an inch thick, then you have too much fat, and need to lose weight. A more precise way, if you are mathematically inclined, is to use the formula of Dr John Garrow of Northwick Park Hospital in London. You may need a pocket calculator, for Dr Garrow divides the weight in kilograms by the square of the height in metres. The resulting number for a normal weight in men should be between 20 and 25, and for women between 19 and 24. For example, a man 5 ft 10 in tall (1.78 m), weighing 12st 4lb (78kg), would calculate as follows:

For the square of the height, multipy $1.78 \times 1.78 = 3.18$. Divide the weight by this number, divide 78 by 3.18 = 24.60

As 24.60 is within the normal range for men, he need not worry about his weight.

Try this method using your unclothed weight, and if your total is higher than 25, whether you are male or female, seriously consider taking off those extra pounds. Aim for, say, 23, but be happy if you reach 25.

How to lose weight successfully

Before you even start to think about losing weight I must make one important point clear. High blood pressure is *not* an emergency condition which is going to destroy your life within days of its diagnosis. So do *not* embark upon a crash diet to take off many pounds very quickly. You have plenty of time to reduce the weight, sensibly and slowly, and enjoy yourself as you do so.

It is important that you do enjoy your new way of eating for you are setting yourself a pattern for the rest of your life. The aim, remember, is not only to lose weight, but to keep it stable once it is in the normal range. If you don't enjoy your new eating habits, you will eventually revert to your old ones, and put the lost weight back on. Nineteen of every twenty slimmers regain their original weights, and even more, within a year after losing weight.

The other key to steady and permanent weight loss is to keep your eating habits 'normal'. This means avoiding diets that involve lists of food to take and others to avoid, all marked with calorie levels that you must count each day. You cannot keep up either specialized diets or calorie counts for ever, unless you are particularly anxious about your health (another thing to avoid if you have high blood pressure). You will be bound to fall by the wayside, eventually.

Instead, make sure you have well-cooked, tasty, varied meals, and leave the dining table happily satisfied, but never bloated. And stick to the following easy rules:

1 Have a good breakfast every day, even if it means rising half an hour earlier to do so. In years of talking to fat people in my family practice, I have found very few who ever take breakfast. Most say they have no time for a morning meal – because they get up too late for more than a cup of tea or coffee before going to work, or simply because they can't face food first thing in the morning.

The breakfast should provide the energy to see you through the day. For instance, as part of a high fibre diet, a mixed cereal such as muesli is a good starter, as is porridge. Follow that with grilled bacon, or a poached or boiled egg, or a kipper, and take toast and coffee or tea as you wish. You will go to work feeling good, and are less likely to be tempted by biscuits or cakes at the mid-morning break.

It may well be that you can't face breakfast because you habitually have a large evening meal. Having your main meal in the evening is just asking to put on weight, especially nowadays when usually the only activity afterwards is watching television, then sleeping. That is a sure way to convert what you have eaten into fat stores, while dulling your appetite for a healthy breakfast next morning.

2 Start your new eating habits by missing out your evening meal: tonight, if possible. Instead, settle your hunger, and help yourself to sleep, with a warm milk drink about half an hour before bed. Set your alarm for half an hour earlier than usual, and you will wake up ravenous, and ready for that good breakfast, which you will have plenty of time to cook.

3 Go on as you have started. The whole point of this change of eating habits – don't call it a diet, as this suggests that you can abandon it after you have reached your desired weight – is that it is a change for life, one that you will grow to like and not wish to abandon for your former fattening ways.

4 Examine what you eat, how varied it is, and how it is cooked. Don't pay too much attention, yet, to *how much* you eat. Most diets restrict the amounts of food you eat, and starve you into losing weight, and that means eventually you will give way to temptation. Instead, include in your menu as many vegetable and salad foods as you can. Add as much fresh fruit as you wish and make it a rule almost always to choose it in preference to puddings. Almost, because you will have earned, and enjoy an occasional small 'reward' when you find you have lost a little more.

5 Pale meats such as poultry and fish are less fattening than steaks and beef, so choose them most of the time, rather than the red meats.

6 Don't eat between meals. Take only coffee or tea at between-meal breaks, and resist the buns and biscuits.

That will leave you better able to eat your lunch, which should be light and tasty, and to enjoy your one-course evening meal.

7 How you cook is important. Grill, rather than fry. Boil or bake potatoes rather than roast or fry them, and eat the skins – they provide extra roughage. Lightly steam vegetables, so that they are just cooked, and if you are still hungry at the end of the meal, eat a little more vegetable, rather than a sweet or fatty dessert. Or eat a piece of fresh fruit.

8 Do recognize that eating too well, or unwisely, at meal times, is not the only way you can get fat. Between-meal snacks, and drinks – particularly if with milk and sugar – will make you put on stones over the years, even if you eat reasonably at mealtimes. The usual cry of the overweight – that 'I don't eat much' – is from people who conveniently forget the numerous snacks they consume all through the day. The same goes for alcoholic drinks, all of which can cause you to put on weight – a 'beer-belly' is the commonest example, but there are just as many paunches resulting from gin and tonic, wine or whisky.

9 Finally, your eating habits are only part of the story of how you became fat. The other half is exercise, or rather lack of it. For years, you have eaten too much for your energy expenditure. You can resolve that by eating less, or expending more energy. It is usually best to do both. Most fat people seem to avoid physical exercise as much as they can. As you start your new life of eating for health and a lower blood pressure, resolve to exercise more, too. It will do you no harm, and probably do enormous good, provided you set about it sensibly. A guide as to how best to do this is given in Chapter 6.

After some weeks of the new life-style, your capacity for food will fall, and you will wonder how it was that you could have eaten such large quantities. Once you are at that stage, you have succeeded: you should not backslide again. Do be wary, however, of starting to eat more again, especially at crises in your life. Many people eat to overcome worries, so guard against this trap.

Crash diets and commercial aids Advice on how to slim appears in many magazines, and some are devoted to slimming. Indeed, the continuing popularity of the subject suggests that the advice is either not taken or it is incorrect! If you have high blood pressure and are too heavy, don't look for a solution via a crash diet, or one of the commercialized diets. If they don't allow you to eat normal foods, they are a waste of time.

The other waste of time, and definitely not recommended for fat people with high blood pressure, are drugs to help you slim. They only work for a short time, if at all, and many have undesirable side-effects, including a mental 'boost' effect that the user can become dependent upon. Doctors in the United Kingdom now rarely prescribe them, and would be very unhappy to give them to patients with high blood pressure, as they can induce anxiety and tension, the very symptoms to be avoided.

On the other hand, some people find sharing their problems with others similarly affected very helpful, and self-help clubs for slimmers have been very successful. However, I am wary of groups who 'fine' members for failing to lose weight, as this can be distressing and worrying – two reactions that should be avoided in anyone seriously attempting to lose weight, but especially so in people with high blood pressure. A group that works in a pleasant, supportive and encouraging atmosphere, rather than by bullying, is better in the long run.

Restricting salt

The part played by salt in producing high blood pressure

was suggested as long ago as 1904, when doctors for the first time closely related the highly salted food of six patients with their high blood pressure, and showed that the blood pressure fell when they ate food with little or no salt. It was not until the 1940s, however, that low salt diets were generally used in medicine to treat dangerously high blood pressure. Almost completely restricted to rice, fruit and sugar, the diets were very unpleasant to maintain for more than short periods, and although very effective in reducing high blood pressures, were abandoned when drugs that could control the pressure almost as well were introduced.

Recently, the vogue for restricting salt in the food of people with high blood pressure has returned, after doctors in Britain and Australia found that they could lower hypertension and make their patients feel better, just by eliminating any added salt from their diet. Patients were told not to add any salt to their food, in the cooking or at table, and to avoid foods to which salt had been added in their processing. Compared with other patients with similar levels of blood pressure, treated in the same way by the same doctors, but without the low-salt advice, the low-salt group maintained their blood pressures at lower levels and it became possible to cut down on the numbers and doses of their blood-pressure-lowering drugs.

Those put on the low salt diet were expected not to like their new cuisine. Instead they felt happier and healthier, and began to enjoy the subtleties of taste that the withdrawal of salt allowed them to experience. It appeared that their previous use of salt had blunted their sense of other tastes.

Simply the amount of salt sprinkled on food may increase blood pressure in some people. Strangely, the amount swallowed in this way appears to depend not on a liking for a particular amount of salt – but on the size of the holes in the salt cellar! People tend to sprinkle salt on their food before tasting it, and shake the salt cellar for the same time, whether the salt pours out from large holes or sprinkles out from small ones.

In 1983, the National Advisory Committee on Nutrition Education (NACNE), the first British Government body in forty years to give practical advice on diet goals, proposed as one of its first priorities that people should reduce their salt intake by a quarter. NACNE recognized, however, that food cooked with less or no salt might not become acceptable overnight. It suggested that greater use of other flavourings such as herbs, spices and lemon juice, would be helpful, and asked the food industry to explore ways of reducing the salt content of nearly all processed foods.

The anti-salt lobby believe that today's food contains ten to fifteen times as much salt as was eaten by our ancestors. So returning to the so-called 'low' salt diet simply takes us back to the salt levels for which our bodies were designed. Other experts are not so sure. They say that the definitive research proving the benefits of lowering salt intake has yet to be done. Also, other studies have not confirmed the initial British and Australian studies, three failing to find any reduction in blood pressure in people taking a low salt diet.

Just as important, the original studies did not look for any possible harm accruing from the long term adoption of a low salt diet. The anti-salt restriction group point out that some laboratory rats even raise their blood pressures when deprived of salt. Is it possible, they ask, that some people could react similarly? Several hypertension experts put their views on this subject strongly, in a letter to *The Lancet* in 1984, as follows:

We are concerned with the way in which this important issue is being handled. The idea that salt in the diet has some possible value is totally ignored. Instead some are even suggesting that salt is a general poison like alcohol or tobacco. The usual scientific standards for weighing evidence and giving advice, now well established in drug development and prescribing, seem to have been forgotten in an evangelical crusade to present a simplistic view of the evidence which will prove attractive to the media.

There is an urgent need for properly conducted scientific studies of the effect of prolonged alterations in salt intake in order to assess the consequences of such advice. Some individuals may be helped by salt restriction, some may be harmed. We should be prepared to devote at least the same time, trouble and money to analysis of the national diet as we insist is devoted to the analysis of drug toxicity.

Scientific studies *have* been completed since 1984 (see page 96, 'The salt saga – the final word'), but doctors can still not be sure that people with high blood pressure should always be advised to restrict their salt intake.

To cut down on salt added to the food after cooking is almost certainly harmless, and may well do some good for your blood pressure. If you find the taste too bland, use pepper or other spices instead. You may find, as the weeks pass, that your ability to taste flavours in foods improves greatly now that your taste buds are no longer overwhelmed by salt.

You will probably benefit from cutting out foods that are heavily salted in their preparation. Among them are:

salted butter, cheese, biscuits, all foods made with self-raising flour, tomato ketchups and sauces, soya sauces, pickles, crisps, all forms of tinned meats and sausages, ham, sardines, and smoked fish and meats. The popular hamburger and chips are loaded with salt.

Deep-frozen, fresh foods are the only preserved foods you can depend on to be low in salt.

However, there are two very good reasons why no one with high blood pressure should embark on a low salt diet without first discussing it with his or her doctor:

1 The change in blood pressure needs to be monitored so that any further steps can be taken, such as lowering the dose of drugs, or changing them according to the subsequent fall in pressure – if it occurs.
2 Some drug treatments actually work better if you keep up your salt intake.

If after two months or so of a low salt intake, your blood pressure has not improved, and your drug dosage cannot be substantially reduced, there is no point in carrying on with the low salt regime – unless you simply feel better. It is more important to enjoy your food than to persevere with a diet that you may dislike and has no benefits.

The fat debate

The argument about salt is nothing compared with that about the sort of fats we eat. Basically there are two forms of fats – those of animal origin, known as the 'hard' or 'saturated' fats, and those from vegetables, known as the 'soft' or 'polyunsaturated' fats. There are certain exceptions to these rules – some vegetable fats and oils veer towards the hard side, and fish and marine animal oils act in the body much more like the soft than the hard fats.

The accepted wisdom at the moment is that the 'good' fats and oils come from vegetables and fish, and the 'bad' fats and oils from animals, particularly those with red, rather than pale meat. Beef and mutton, for example, have more hard fat, pound for pound, than poultry.

It is said that the hard fats are bad, because people with high levels of them in their circulation have a higher than normal death rate from diseases of the blood vessels, such as heart attacks and strokes. However, it has never been proved that reducing the fats in the circulation by diet or drugs will definitely prevent such deaths.

Despite this lack of proof, if you have high blood

pressure, it seems only sensible to cut down your intake of animal fats, and replace them with the apparently safer foods containing the 'soft' oils and fats. In the following table of some of the foods we most commonly eat, the 'good' foods are on the left, the 'bad' foods on the right. Chicken and turkey are somewhere in between. Fish and fish oil, though strictly not in the 'soft' category by chemical structure, are definitely in the 'good' column because they appear to protect against, rather than promote, blood vessel disease.

Low hard fat foods	*High hard fat foods*
Beer	Cheeses
Cereals	Cream and ice-cream
Cottage cheese	Duck
Flour	Eggs
Fruit	Goose
Oils (vegetable)	Hard margarine
Skimmed milk	Lard
Soft margarine	Meats
Spaghetti and other pastas	Milk
Yoghurt	Suet

This is only a guide. It does *not* mean that we should exclude all the foods on the right, and eat only those on the left. A good variety of foods is needed for a balanced diet: the important thing is not to eat too much!

Importance of fibre

Fibre has also attracted much recent interest, and the evidence for everyone – not just those with high blood pressure – to eat food containing plenty of fibre every day is very good. People with a high fibre intake have a lower risk of heart attacks than people eating food containing very little fibre – it is said because fibre directly lowers the blood pressure.

High fibre foods are wholemeal bread, potatoes, peas and beans – yes, even the much abused baked bean – and cereals. Eating them gives a 'full-up' feeling that lasts, and they contain many nutrients while having a low concentration of those fattening calories. They also help to give bulk to your motions, making constipation and straining to open your bowels less likely. All in all, fibre is very good for people with high blood pressure, and is highly recommended.

Sugar

Sugar is yet another controversial foodstuff. Among the food experts its reputation varies from that of the devil incarnate to something that simply provides too many calories and rots your teeth. There is no positive proof that eating sugar will affect your blood vessels or your blood pressure, except that, if you are overweight, its high calorie value will not help you to slim. On the whole, if you are not overweight and not diabetic, sugar in moderation does not seem to be very harmful – though you may have to visit your dentist more often than you would like.

Restricting alcohol

The effects of moderate amounts of alcohol on high blood pressure may surprise you. They may actually help to bring it *down* – but it depends very much on how you define 'moderate'. One or two standard drinks a day – a standard drink is a glass of wine, sherry or other fortified wine, a small measure of a spirit, or a half pint of beer – will probably do no harm. The benefit seems to come from alcohol's action in opening up the small blood vessels in the skin, thereby lowering the resistance to the flow of blood, and lowering the diastolic pressure. However, the harm starts to mount up if you drink every day to a level of more than twenty standard drinks a week.

Even small amounts of alcoholic drink, especially when taken with a soft drink 'mixer', have a high energy value, which has to be counted in a weight-losing diet, but the real danger of alcohol is when you start taking too much. Heavy drinking, even if it does not reach the stage of alcoholism, very definitely shortens life. Anything over fifteen to twenty standard drinks a week may raise your blood pressure, and heavy drinking directly poisons the heart. In countries where alcohol is a serious problem, as in France and Sweden, heavy drinking is the single most common cause of early death in men in their forties.

If you have high blood pressure, you need not become a teetotaller; but you must restrict your intake to one or two drinks at most each day, and try to spend three days each week without any alcohol.

The case against smoking

If you have high blood pressure, you are crazy if you smoke. It is as simple as that. Just consider the effects that smoking has on your circulation and heart. By inhaling cigarette smoke directly into your lungs, bypassing the normal filtering, warming and moistening air-conditioning that the nose is designed to impose on all the air you breathe, you take into your body three highly potent poisons: tars, nicotine, and carbon monoxide. We will take them one by one, to look at their relevance to high blood pressure.

Tars

All the poisons in the tars have not yet been fully identified. This is not surprising, because there are thousands of them, and most are complex chemicals that will damage any living tissue with which they come into contact. As smokers suck them directly into the lungs bypassing the biological traps set for them in the nose, throat, and larynx (the voice box), the delicate airways deep in the lungs are directly exposed to them. Of those already identified and tested in animals, many have been shown to cause cancers, and some affect other systems in the body, including the circulation. Just for the tars alone, smoking can seriously harm people with high blood pressure.

Nicotine

Worse, however, from the point of view of hypertension, are the effects of nicotine. If a camera is focused down a microscope on to one of the small blood vessels in the skin of someone who has not smoked for a few days, then he or she starts to smoke a cigarette, within a minute, you can see the blood flow slow, as the vessel narrows in reaction to the nicotine absorbed.

This reaction happens not just in the skin, but all over the body, in the heart and the brain, as well as in all other vital organs. The result is that the blood pressure rises, though only as long as the cigarette lasts. Smoking does not cause sustained high blood pressure, but the most severe and lethal form of high blood pressure occurs far more often in smokers than in non-smokers.

And lighting up a cigarette, with its sudden surge of nicotine in the coronary arteries, may just be the last straw which causes sudden death in the person whose heart is already teetering on the edge of failure. Who knows? For the sudden cramping narrowing it is known to cause in these vessels that feed the heart with oxygen has relaxed again by the time of the post mortem examination.

Carbon monoxide

The carbon monoxide in cigarette smoke (it is the gas that used to be the cause of death in 'head in the oven' suicides in the days before natural gas) is more subtle, but just as lethal. Smokers of twenty cigarettes a day are constantly deprived of the use of about a sixth of their oxygen-carrying red blood cells, because these are 'crippled' by the gas. More than that, the heart muscle (this also has an unfortunate affinity for combining with carbon monoxide), works far less efficiently because of the presence of this poison.

The result of all this is that cigarette smoking is linked with much higher than normal risks of early death from heart attacks and strokes – the same risks that you run if your blood pressure is not kept under good control. If you have both high blood pressure and you smoke, the risks are multiplied, perhaps as much as four times or more.

Even if your blood pressure is normal there are good reasons for not smoking. If it is high, then you need to ensure the best efficiency from all the elements of your circulation: clean lungs, untainted with tar, so that you obtain the maximum of oxygen; open blood vessels for fast flow of blood at low pressure, unaffected by nicotine; and red blood cells and heart muscles working at maximum efficiency, free of carbon monoxide poisoning. If you want that, and surely you do, then you must not smoke at all. It is not a question of cutting down, but of cutting them out, altogether.

When you do stop, the benefits are immediate. You lose the carbon monoxide within a day, and the effects of the nicotine after a week or two. The lungs take longer to get rid of the tar, but after about six months your risk of developing a lung tumour has dropped to the same as if you had never smoked. After a year of non-smoking your extra risk of a heart attack has dropped considerably, but it takes about ten years for that to equal the risk of someone who has never smoked. These are big incentives to stop as soon as possible.

How to stop smoking

Stopping smoking is not as difficult as it sounds. You may do it as General de Gaulle did – by announcing to all your friends that you have done it in such a public way that you would be ashamed to be caught again with a cigarette in your mouth. Most, however, need a lot more support than just your own will power. So ask for the support of your family and friends in not offering you cigarettes; better still, ask them to stop with you. At least they should not smoke when in your company. Make things a little easier for yourself by choosing to stop at a time when you are least stressed – perhaps on holiday, or at the start of a long weekend. Don't attempt it in the middle of a worrying week at work.

People who feel they can't stop often change to a pipe, thinking that it carries less risk. Perhaps that is true of people who have always smoked a pipe, as they rarely inhale, but the cigarette smoker finds it difficult not to inhale, and may even worsen things by changing. So, if you want to quit tobacco, throw away the idea of a pipe, too.

Often, the worst problem starts with the withdrawal of nicotine from your bloodstream. You become irritable, feel unwell, cannot concentrate, and greatly desire a cigarette. Try to hold out, because the worst will soon pass, and you will begin to feel much better within a day or two. Some people are never completely without the desire to start again, but can manage to control the urge. The following aids are recommended:

Nicotine chewing gum can help you to get through this early stage. After years of argument, it has been accepted in the British National Health Service as a treatment to help patients stop smoking. It replaces the lost nicotine, reducing the withdrawal symptoms as the body gets rid of the other chemicals from the smoke. You can then gradually cut down on the gum.

Graduated filter cigarettes (called MD4 in Britain) are another way of easing yourself off the habit. You start by smoking your cigarettes in the first of four see-through cigarette holders which traps a small portion of the tars. Just seeing how much extra muck would have gone into your lungs if you had not used the holder is enough to make you continue using the filters.

As you progress to the other three holders, which trap progressively more and more tars, and are more and more impressive in their collections of disgusting debris after each cigarette, your resolve to stop is strengthened further, until you stop altogether. Some people stick on the last filter, which is better than nothing, but they would be better to stop altogether. After all, the filters do not lessen the amount of carbon monoxide they are inhaling.

Whichever way you choose, the determination to stop has to come from you. You now know why it is madness to continue, and if you make the immediate decision always to respond, without the slightest second thought, with 'no, thank you' to the offer of a cigarette, you are well on your way to success. Many millions of Britons have stopped smoking in the last five years; the consumption of cigarettes has fallen by twenty per cent. There is every reason for you, if you are a smoker, to join them.

5

How to Handle Stress

One of the most useless pieces of advice ever given to anyone, with any disease, is to 'take it easy and relax'. First, it doesn't explain how to follow that advice – so it worries people more, and makes them *less* relaxed. Second, most people who are worried and under stress are like that because they see no way round their problems. They have to solve their problems *before* they can relax. Third, and probably most important, there is no guarantee that relaxing will improve their medical condition, or proof that their anxiety was the cause of their illness. If they relax, and are still ill, they are still at square one, and have an added resentment against the person who gave them the foolish advice!

So, before rushing into the effects of stress and anxiety on high blood pressure, let us take a look at a few definitions. For example, what do we mean by stress, and is there any definite link between stress and high blood pressure? The very word hypertension suggests that emotional tension may be involved, but the proof of a direct link between the two is tenuous, and the benefits of relaxation in lowering blood pressure are not as clear as, say, those of penicillin in curing infections.

Defining stress

Stress is any exceptional outside pressure on you to which you must react, mentally and physically. The stress can be mental, as when a combination of financial, employment-related, emotional, marital and other family worries crowd in on you, or physical, as with a too-demanding, exhausting or repetitive job. Often it is a combination of both.

Whatever the cause, it has far-reaching effects on your

body systems, setting your circulation's 'throttle' at a higher than normal level, and possibly – but not always – producing high blood pressure.

Individual reactions to stress

From the many studies of blood pressure in large numbers of people picked at random from apparently normal populations, it seems that stress itself rarely initiates persistent high blood pressure. You must be already the type to respond to stress with sustained high blood pressure before you are exposed to it. Others exposed to stress, mental or physical, may briefly show a blood pressure slightly higher than normal, but this is not sustained even if the stress remains.

Some idea of the proportion of people who fit the two groups can be gauged from reports of disasters in the United States. Two weeks after a huge nitrate explosion in Texas City in 1948, more than half the survivors had diastolic blood pressures above 95 mm Hg. A flood in Buffalo Creek, in the early 1950s, appears to have induced high blood pressure that has been sustained in some survivors to this day. It is known also that battle produces high blood pressure and this may last for two months or more after removal from the combat zone.

More prolonged, if less dramatic, stress has also been linked with hypertension. Unemployment and low income, and living in areas of severe social deprivation are all associated with higher rates of, and deaths from, high blood pressure, although it is difficult to rule out from these studies other possible causes for the hypertension, such as diet and family history of the disease.

Stress affects blood pressure even in childhood. A study of schoolchildren in the Philippines showed that blood pressures were higher in children who were struggling academically than in those who were in the top academic group and doing well.

Just as relevant to this study are the figures for groups of people who tend to have *lower* blood pressures than the rest of the population. They include, perhaps not unexpectedly, regular attenders at church. Presumably they have a higher authority on whom to load their stress! Paradoxically, they also include male prison inmates, surely among the most stressed people in any community.

Personality

If different people react differently to stress, what is the origin of the difference? Is it to be found in the personality of the individual? In 1939, Dr Franz Alexander, an American researcher in psychosomatic medicine, suggested that people with high blood pressure had strong hostile tendencies which they suppressed and turned inwards, instead of expressing them outwardly.

This inward expression of anger, Dr Alexander proposed, produced a rise in blood pressure that became permanent. Today's view is that this may hold good for only a few hypertensives, and that the vast majority have the same spread of personality characteristics as the general population. The difficulty in trying to analyse the personalities of people already known to have the disease is that the disease itself may have changed the personality, through its effects on the nervous system, so making any assessment of the pre-high blood pressure personality impossible.

However, examples of the different reactions to stress in people with normal blood pressure and those with high blood pressure do suggest that once you *are* hypertensive, you tend to react differently to stress.

In 1971 a Dr J.D. Sapira and his colleagues showed two films to groups of people with high blood pressure and with normal blood pressure. One film showed a doctor interviewing a patient in a rude, disinterested manner, the other showed a different doctor, who was considerate, kind, friendly and communicated well with the patient.

When asked to comment, the people with normal blood pressures were quick to see the differences between the two interviews (and showed very small changes in heart rate and blood pressure while watching). The hypertensives, on the other hand, did not comment on the differences between the doctors' attitudes, and even denied seeing them. Yet their blood pressures and heart rates rose much more than those of the normal pressure group!

Effects of suppressed emotions

American women college students with high blood pressure, asked to act out their responses to stressful situations, had difficulty in expressing emotions such as fear and anger. Their colleagues with normal blood pressures had no such problems.

This apparent confirmation of suppressed anger or emotion as a factor in hypertensive patients is supported by the 1977 findings of Dr M. Esler and colleagues. They found that patients whose high blood pressure was linked with suppressed hostility had higher than normal levels in their blood of the chemicals known to raise blood pressure, noradrenaline and renin (see Chapter 2). Could this be a stepwise process, the suppressed anger leading to the higher production of the chemicals, and then to the high blood pressure? If so, then altering patients' reactions to stress, by persuading them either not to react with anger, or at least not to suppress it, may prevent the blood pressure rise.

This is the basis of all self-help advice on stress to hypertension sufferers. Change the way you look at things, so that you do not immediately react with anger or anxiety; and if you find that you are reacting in these ways, consciously try to wipe them from your mind. Relaxation and meditation are the traditional ways of doing this.

Personality types

Much has been written on Type A and Type B personalities. The Type As are aggressive, ambitious people who work longer hours than most, thrive on competition, and play hard, too. Their families are relatively neglected in favour of business commitments. They smoke, drink, and eat well – usually too well – and when they have time for their hobbies, they love to compete even then. A game of squash is never really enjoyed unless they have won, and if they jog, they time their run, rather than enjoy the exercise and the view.

The Type Bs are happy to carry on in routine jobs, looking on them as a necessary interval between the times they like most, spent with the family. Their real interest in life is anything from stamp collecting or walking in the countryside, to simply watching the television or reading. Type Bs will never be promoted to the heights, but are still invaluable employees; they tend to have happier home lives and it is claimed that, on average, they live longer than the Type As, because they are less likely to have a coronary thrombosis.

All this may seem like advice for the Type As among you to become more like Type Bs. Yet that isn't strictly the case. Because, although the Type As are more likely to die young from heart attacks if they do not 'take things easier', high blood pressure does not seem to be to blame. Type Bs are just as likely to develop high blood pressure as Type As. Perhaps under that placid, apparently unruffled exterior, there are hidden emotions that should be released!

Ways of dealing with stress

The following advice is applicable to everyone with high blood pressure, whether you recognize yourself as closer to a Type A or to a Type B person, whatever the known cause of your particular type of high blood pressure, and irrespective of how severe it is. None of these tips for dealing with stress can harm you, and any one of them may help to bring your pressure down. Even if it does not, and you still need drugs for complete control, you will almost certainly feel some benefit.

Face up to yourself
If you have high blood pressure, try to make an objective review of your own personality, your life-style, your worries and fears, and how you react to them. This may be the first time you have faced them, coolly, and logically. If it is, that in itself may show that you have suppressed some truths about yourself, from yourself.

The purpose of such a review is not to learn how to avoid meeting stress – for example, by leaving your job for an easier one – but to learn how to face up to the ones you meet in your present environment. Stress is not bad in itself, it is the way we react to it that can cause problems. Of course, too much stress in your life cannot be good, but you should feel able to enjoy some challenge in your work and leisure. This is especially true of young people, whose initiatives and ability to work hard and to progress in a career can only be developed by being faced with stressful situations. Provided they see it in this light, they will come to no harm.

Excessive stress shows itself in easily recognized physical symptoms:

● The commonest is the tension headache that feels like a vice being applied over the surface of the skull, from stiff muscles in the back of the neck to the forehead and eyebrows. The eyes, too, may feel tense and ache.
● You may sleep badly.
● You may have palpitations.
● You may have bouts of diarrhoea alternating with constipation.
● You may lose your appetite.

Any of these symptoms should warn you that stress is getting on top, and needs to be approached in a different way. Whether the stress is related to anxieties at work or at home, ask yourself the following questions:

- Am I coping with my everyday responsibilities?
- If not, how can I change my life so that I can?
- Who can I ask to help me change in the right direction?
- Am I suppressing feelings, of anger, fear, or worry, that I should have openly expressed to the person who can do something about them, or at least help me to share them?
- Am I neglecting one important area of my life by devoting too much time to another?
- If so, how can I take practical steps to change that?
- Do I relax enough, at any time of each day, and forget my worries?
- If not, when can I spare the time to do so, and what should I do?

You will notice that the answers to all these questions need action from *you* and not your doctor, or even your family or colleagues at work. You have to take the first step towards a better approach to stress; you are on your own until you have done so. From then on, others can help you.

Let us assume that you have taken all the right decisions:

- Your too-heavy work load has been discussed with your boss, and you have an assistant.
- You have delegated that next sales trip to your deputy so that you can spend more time with your long-suffering family.
- You found that your bank manager could help you over that financial trouble which has kept your awake for weeks.
- You have taken time to have that long-needed fatherly chat with your teenage daughter.

What next? Do you still feel tense and find it difficult to relax? If you do, there is no need to feel that you are in any way exceptional – a 1976 survey of American families showed that only 18 per cent felt they had no need to reduce the stress in their lives, and there is no reason to suppose that there is less stress today. Try one of the techniques in relaxation outlined below – choose the one that most appeals to you and it will almost certainly be of help.

Progressive muscle relaxation

This is the most simple of the modern techniques, and one with which it is easy to start. It has been used to ease phobias, or unreasonable fears about everyday things, and has been claimed also to bring down blood pressure. Just lie down in a quiet room, and systematically tense and relax the different groups of muscles in your body, concentrating on each in turn until you have covered them all. You can start and finish where you like, say with the big back muscles, moving on to the neck, then the shoulders, the arms and fingers, then to the thighs, legs, feet and toes, and so on.

The technique is described in detail in *You Must Relax* by E. Jacobsen, published by McGraw-Hill, New York, in 1978.

Hypnotic relaxation

This is induced by suggestions of relaxing muscle tone after you have been put into a hypnotic state by a qualified practitioner. In a series of sessions, you can be taught to put yourself 'under', and pass into a deeply relaxed state. The sessions focus on different triggers to help you relax: one may be a feeling of heaviness in the limbs, another a feeling of warmth. With experience, you learn to recognize the ways most effective for you to become completely relaxed.

Meditation

The practice of meditation to induce relaxation, and incidentally to reduce blood pressure, stems from the East, largely from Yoga and Transcendental Meditation (TM).

Yoga relaxation exercises concentrate on taking up particular physical postures and control of breathing. Transcendental meditation involves you in twice daily sessions, sitting in a comfortable upright position, breathing slowly and peacefully, and repeating a special sound or word, called a mantra.

Both are fairly simple relaxation techniques, but some teachers complicate their use with mystical and philosophical ideas from Eastern religions which can be off-putting for the average Western man or woman. This is a pity because the relaxant effect of the exercises does not appear to depend at all on acceptance of the teacher's religious views! Many evening institutions run Yoga classes, so you may well find one within easy reach and can try it out for yourself.

The relaxation response

An American doctor, H. Benson, has adapted the TM techniques to a more Westernized relaxation system, which he calls the 'relaxation response'. It has the following instructions:

1 Sit quietly and comfortably.
2 Close your eyes.
3 Relax all your muscles, beginning with your feet, and continuing up to your legs, torso, arms, shoulders, neck and face, just by letting the muscles go limp.
4 Breathe rhythmically through your nose. Be aware of your breathing. As you breathe out, say the word 'one' silently.
5 Continue for 20 minutes. Then complete the session by sitting quietly for a few minutes.
6 Do not worry about whether you are successful at

67

attaining a deep level of relaxation. Maintain a passive attitude and permit relaxation to occur at its own pace. When distracting thoughts occur, ignore them and keep repeating the word 'one'.

7 Practise these exercises twice daily.

This programme has the merit of being very easy to conduct yourself, and does appear to help lower high blood pressure in some people. It must be stressed, however, that as with all these techniques, it is complementary, and not an alternative, to the orthodox management of high blood pressure. If it allows your doctor to reduce your prescribed drugs, so much the better, but under no circumstances should you reduce the dose yourself. Do tell your doctor what you are doing. He will almost certainly encourage you, take special interest in the progress of your pressure as the months go by, and change or reduce your prescription as and when he feels this is advisable.

Biofeedback
This technique was designed to help people consciously to identify bodily measurements not normally under conscious control – such as skin temperature, heart rate and blood pressure and learn to control them at will. The person undergoing biofeedback is given an apparatus to measure the system, and taught how to use it so that he or she can watch how the pressure responds to 'thinking it down'.

It is not known how simply thinking about lowering one's own blood pressure can produce the desired response, but there is no doubt that it works for some people. The best-known system of biofeedback control of high blood pressure was developed by Dr Chandra Patel, in 1977. She asks patients to lie comfortably on a couch, then to relax their bodies in a systematic way, muscle group by muscle group, while they concentrate on control of their breathing, silently repeating the word 'relax' to themselves as they do so.

Their biofeedback aid is not strictly a measure of blood pressure, but a small wire device which measures the electrical voltage in the skin, the muscles or even the brain waves. The device gives off a sound with a pitch directly related to the electrical activity – the higher the activity, the higher the pitch. As the activity decreases, so the sound lowers in pitch. Patients are encouraged to 'think the pitch down', because as the electrical activity falls, they are more relaxed and their blood pressure usually falls also.

Once Dr Patel's patients have become used to the system, they are encouraged to continue their relaxation exercises twice daily at home. They are shown films about relaxation and biofeedback, and encouraged with great enthusiasm. One extra instruction is to use everyday occurrences to stimulate extra relaxation exercises – such as to check for any signs of muscle tension whenever they come to a red traffic light, or have to use a telephone, or need to look at the time, or whenever the doorbell rings or they have to ring a doorbell.

After twelve weeks of such training, Dr Patel's patients find their blood pressures have been reduced by as much as 28/15 mm Hg, a very significant fall, and well worth their efforts. The measurements are made at the start of each relaxation session, and not at the finish, so that the results can fairly be considered a change in their average blood pressures, and not simply the transient result of a good relaxation session.

Anyone could follow the example of the Patel method. The instrument for measuring the skin voltage is probably not essential – the real benefit comes from the time spent relaxing, and the frequent reminders during the day to check for the encroachment of tension in the muscles.

Natural methods – not drugs
The key to the success of all these relaxation techniques is to persist in practising them, day after day, at home, as often as is convenient, and even, when there is time to

spare, at work. Once you are into the habit of consciously relaxing the different muscle groups, it becomes easy and virtually second nature. While they do not work for everyone, in the sense that they will not always bring the blood pressure down, they should always make you *feel* better, and that in itself is a bonus. Everyone who feels the need to relax at some time in any day, and that must mean all of us, could benefit.

One last comment about relaxation for the patient with high blood pressure. You may be tempted to ask for tranquillizers or sedatives to ease your tension and help you relax. Do not be surprised if your doctor refuses to prescribe them. Tranquillizers would only complicate the already complex reactions in your circulatory system, and might interfere with the drugs prescribed to bring down the pressure.

Tranquillizers are *not* a treatment for high blood pressure, and only disguise your reaction to stress, without solving the underlying problems. So avoid taking them unless there is a good reason for them – the only one that springs to mind is a neurotic anxiety state thought to have been present before the start of the high blood pressure, and completely unrelated to it. That must be very rare.

6

Exercise – The Good and the Bad

One of the most remarkable changes in our society in recent years has been the upsurge – some might say the mania – for exercise. Who could have imagined, only a few years ago, that 10,000 people would take part in marathons in many cities around Britain, every year? Or that millions of people would desert the spectator sports and television sets to do their own thing, in athletics, squash, tennis, and a host of other energetic occupations?

The switch to more active leisure pursuits is no passing fad, but a real change in people's habits that can only be welcomed, along with the concern for better eating habits, and the fall in tobacco consumption.

For the person with high blood pressure, the change is of particular benefit. For the correct kind of exercise will help to re-set your pressure at a lower level, even though the act of exercise itself will temporarily raise it. Getting yourself fit helps your circulation, improves the blood flow through your muscles, and improves the efficiency of your heart – all excellent improvements for anyone with high blood pressure. If you are overweight, and most people start off with some flab, the right sort of exercise will trim you down and firm you up, not only making you look and feel better, but reducing the workload of the heart.

If you need convincing about the long-term benefits of exercise, the following figures may make you think, though I am not suggesting you should aim for professional status as an athlete!

● A group of long distance skiers in Finland lived, on average, 4.3 years longer than the rest of that country's relatively healthy population.

 Major League Baseball players in the United States between the years 1876 and 1973 tended to live much longer than the general male American population.

 Among British student athletes, runners lived longer than throwers, irrespective of the distance they ran. 57 per cent of the sprinters, 56 per cent of the long-distance runners, but only 34 per cent of the hammer throwers and shot putters reached the age of seventy years, even though most of them stopped their athletic careers after leaving college.

 People who continue their running throughout their lives not only live longer, but have lower blood pressures than the general population of the same age.

However these figures are interpreted, and many will draw different conclusions from them, they all have the same trend – towards dynamic exercise as being good for you. And that applies just as much to the person with high blood pressure as to anyone else.

Having read this far, you are probably reacting to this chapter in one of two ways: 'Good, I really can start some sport again. I thought my high blood pressure had put an end to all that.' Or 'I hate sport and exercise. I always did. Now this fellow's asking me to take it up, when I least feel like it. I wouldn't be seen dead in running kit, and I'm certainly not taking up any form of exercise, so I'll just skip the rest of this chapter.'

Both reactions are quite normal, and the second one is especially understandable. There are plenty of people who see no sense in sports or any more phsyical exercise than absolutely necessary. Nevertheless, if you are one of them, do take the trouble to read on, because the first part of this chapter is intended for you, and advises how you can improve your fitness in fairly undemanding ways.

An active approach to the day

If you are dead set against running, swimming, cycling, or even a brisk walk every day, there are still ways you can stimulate your heart and circulation out of their sluggish rut – because that is what they are in. It is simply a question of re-organizing your day so that you are more active in going about your usual tasks.

Presumably your sum of physical activity consists of a walk out of the house to the car or bus, perhaps driving to a station, and a journey, seated, to work, where you spend the rest of the day sitting down. Then it is home again, to enjoy your evening meal, and sit in your favourite chair to watch television. Not once in the day have you been so much as a little out of breath. And if you look back over the years, it is difficult to remember when you last broke into a run.

Looking at your life like that, it must dawn on you that this is hardly a healthy existence. Just try running up a short flight of stairs, and see how long it takes you to get your breath back. Does it surprise you? If it does, but you are still not convinced that you need to exercise, then at least start to do a little more to make your day more active.

First, what about that journey to work? Do you take your car or the bus less than a mile? If so, why not walk? It will take a little longer, but no more than a quarter of an hour at normal walking speed. You will feel fresher when you get to work, and will take a new interest in your surroundings on the way. You could use different routes from time to time, for added interest. The simple expedient of walking two miles a day – one mile there and back – will start the 'toning up' process.

If your journey is longer than a mile, then at least walk part of the way, then take public transport, so that you can relax for the rest of the journey. A few bus stops, or the distance between two suburban stations, are ideal to start with. There is an extra bonus, in that if you have left your car at home you will be avoiding the blood-pressure-raising stress of driving in the rush hour traffic.

Once you get to work, use the stairs instead of the lift. In fact, make a point of always using the stairs in any building, such as department stores and flats, providing you don't get too much out of breath, and you keep the effort down to three floors. Any higher and you can allow yourself the luxury of the escalator or lift.

In the office, if you are seated all day, get up and walk around every hour or so. It will stretch those cramped muscles, In the lunch hour, take a walk, rather than sit around. You will have more time to do so than before, because you will be eating less!

On the way home, get off the bus one or two stops before your home and walk the rest of the way. After your light evening meal, take a brisk walk if you still feel you have the energy, preferably with company. Your partner will be so happy at your new found energy, she or he will probably be delighted to join you. It could be the start of a new interest in each other's company. A word of advice though – don't make the walk straight to the pub; that may well negate the good that the exercise has done you.

If you have no companion, why not try walking a dog? Dogs need walking, and the very fact that you have one in a house, if you live alone, can lower your blood pressure. Simply sitting stroking a well-loved dog or cat in the comfort of your own home has been shown to lower the blood pressure; and even a cat requires some expenditure of energy, if only to be let in and out at regular intervals.

In the home, try doing without some labour-saving gadgets. The worst is the remote control TV switch. Get rid of it, so that you have to get up and walk over to the set every time you wish to change programmes or switch off. You can probably think of dozens of other small things to do that will keep you out of your chair in the evenings and weekends. After a while, you may even grow to like your new life-style, and wish to expand your energy further.

Graduating to more ambitious exercise

The next step, provided your doctor approves, is to buy a bicycle, or go to the local swimming pool for the first time for years, or maybe take a long country walk. If you have reached this stage, you are well on the way to a fitter life, and you may surprise your doctor on your next visit for a blood pressure check. If you take everything gradually, and talk over your plans with your doctor, you will come to no harm, and start to feel fitter than you have for years. It is often only then that people realize quite how unpleasant it is to be unfit.

You probably wish to curtail your new exercise habit at this stage, and if that is the way you feel, you are perfectly correct to do so. There is no definite proof that taking up a regular sport, such as running, *will* make you any fitter, or bring your blood pressure down any further. If you are keen to take up an active sport or exercise, however, so much the better, provided you don't try to do too much, too soon.

Don't start exercising if you feel unwell in any way. And if, when you start, you have any pain in your chest, neck, upper tummy or back, or feel sick or exhausted, stop at once, and seek medical advice. Usually such symptoms are of minor importance, but they do need checking by your doctor. This particularly applies to people who have had previous heart attacks or know that they have angina, but it is also a good rule for everyone.

Having had a heart attack, however, is by no means a bar to quite strenuous exercise. Provided you have the all-clear from your doctors, you can follow programmes of exercise that can lead to completing marathons – as many Americans and Canadians have found to their delight. Dr T. Kavanagh, who runs a Rehabilitation Centre for heart patients in Toronto, has helped several of his patients to complete marathons. He has a trophy named after him, inscribed 'Dr T. Kavanagh, Supercoach, The World's Sickest Track Club'! Dr Kavanagh bases his advice on careful assessment of each person's condition. There is a graduated programme, beginning in some cases with as little as a one mile walk lasting thirty minutes. Even after graduating to running, his patients are advised not to run faster than a mile in ten minutes.

If you are interested in taking up running, one book to read is *The Complete Book of Running* by James E. Fixx, published by Chatto and Windus. Mr Fixx took up running in his mid-thirties when he weighed nearly 16 stones and was breathing hard after fifty yards. More than anyone else, he was responsible for the popularity of jogging today. He ran for years, getting down to 11 stones. James Fixx died in 1984, in his late fifties, ironically of a heart attack while running. It is difficult to judge, not knowing the man, why he should succumb in this way. He is said to have ignored warning signs, and continued to do too much when he should have slowed down and sought medical advice. He was certainly an enthusiast, to the point of being obsessional about his running. He may well have prolonged his life by many years by taking up running when he did, postponing an inevitable heart attack. No one can ever know. What can be said is that his book is filled with much common sense, despite his own early death.

Older people – the over sixties – should choose the less strenuous sports: walking, swimming and cycling, rather than running or sports involving racquets such as squash or tennis. All hypertensives should avoid taking up serious competitive sport, running against the clock, or team squash where league positions matter to one's colleagues. You should also avoid outdoor exercise in extremes of climate, especially in hot, humid conditions, in which it is impossible to lose heat by sweating. Your blood pressure can climb steeply when running in such weather.

Aside from these warnings, do try to remain energetic – both physically and mentally. All our organs improve with use, and the circulation and brain cells are no exception to that universal rule.

Re-discovering sport and active exercises

It is vital to understand that there are two forms of exercise, one of which should help your blood pressure, the other being possibly dangerous and not to be recommended.

Helpful, dynamic exercise

'Dynamic' exercise is exercise in which your muscles contract to move your body around. Running, walking, swimming, cycling, dancing, aerobics, all fall into this category. You can start on these gradually, and build up your fitness without worrying about your pressure. In the long run, they will help to bring your pressure down. The only word of warning about them is that, if you already have high blood pressure and are receiving medical treatment, take care to discuss with your doctor exactly how much you can do to start with, and build up your activity slowly from that base.

Forms of exercise to avoid

In 'static' or 'isometric' exercise, when the muscle contracts, its length remains the same, but the tension within it rises steeply, giving the explosive power needed, say, in weight lifting, or putting the shot, or pushing furniture around. This type of exercise raises your blood pressure steeply and rapidly, often to very high levels, putting considerable strain on the heart. The change is even greater in people with hypertension than in those with normal blood pressure. Holding your breath while pushing or lifting makes the strain on the heart worse, as it puts up the pressure inside the chest, preventing the blood returning to the heart, at the same time as it is being starved of oxygen. It is easy to understand therefore why hypertensives should avoid such stresses.

This type of stressful exercise is not confined to field sports. You can find yourself in the same situation in an ordinary day, lifting heavy luggage, digging the garden, or shovelling snow, or push-starting the car, or wheeling a barrow, or straining at a constipated stool. Anything that makes you strain and hold your breath should be avoided. Let others do the heavy work; there is usually someone glad to help. If there is no one there at the time, wait until someone comes, or ask for help – don't take chances, or stand on your pride.

Your sex life

Sex is one exercise that most people – even those totally uninterested in any form of athleticism or sport – would be unhappy to give up. Yet few pluck up the courage to ask their doctor directly about this most important aspect of their lives. Some take the decision themselves to stop, in the mistaken belief that it may do them harm. There is a popular fable that the act of sex can 'burst a blood vessel' and induce a stroke, but this is not substantiated by any published research.

In fact, stopping your usual sex life is much more likely to make you worse than better. The stresses and tensions fostered by abstaining will tend to raise your pressure, rather than lower it. During sex, the blood pressure does certainly rise, but it is a rise more than compensated by the relaxation afterwards, and by the emotional balance gained from a good relationship with your partner.

However, one of the complications of the drug treatment of high blood pressure can be a disturbed sex life. Some drugs interfere with erection, and others with ejaculation. Libido may be affected in both sexes. If this is your experience, do not assume that it is due to your blood pressure – *none* of these symptoms are direct results of hypertension. Be sure to mention them to your doctor, as the treatment can be easily changed. How this is done is explained in the next chapter.

7

Prescribed Drugs for High Blood Pressure

The main purpose of this chapter is to describe the types of drugs prescribed by doctors for people with high blood pressure, but it cannot be, and is not intended to be, a catalogue from which you find your own particular treatment, and ignore the others. Drug treatment has been left to the later part of this book to emphasize that it is not the first, or necessarily the major, thought that the doctor has when first deciding to take action against your high blood pressure.

Initial treatment

The very rare case nowadays of a person first attending the doctor with an astronomically high blood pressure, affecting his heart, brain circulation, his kidneys or eyesight, constitutes an emergency for which the only treatment is admission to hospital, and specialist drugs to produce a fast return to normal levels. There is no other reason to look on high blood pressure as a medical emergency: there is always time to take decisions coolly, letting the pressure settle slowly.

White men, black people, and people with a close relative who has been ill or died early from heart disease, are at higher risk than white women, who will be pleased to know that they appear to tolerate higher blood pressures better than men, and have less risk of strokes from the same blood pressure levels. That does not mean to say they can afford to avoid any warning signs (see Chapter 2) but high blood pressure in the higher risk groups may be given extra attention – their doctors may decide to treat the pressure more aggressively, with more powerful drugs.

Bearing in mind the available information about high risk groups, the questions that your doctor runs through, on that first meeting, will follow roughly this pattern:

Is this patient's blood pressure high enough to need treatment? It may not be. A reading of around 150/90 could lead to the perfectly reasonable decision to do nothing, but arrange another appointment, say, in two weeks. Several readings at this level could then lead to discussions about how to bring it down a little without drugs.

If it is high enough to warrant action, should I start treatment with advice only, along the lines of weight loss, life-style changes, relaxation and salt restriction – or should I prescribe drugs from the start? Much depends on the height of the blood pressure, and on whether it remains high when repeated measurements are taken in a less stressful environment than the doctor's surgery or office. A month of weekly measurements taken by the practice nurse at the patient's home may provide the answer.

A fairly standard practice now, based on the results of the Australian and American trials mentioned in Chapter 3, is to take notice of any blood pressure above 140/90, and follow the patient through several readings in the next month. Those who after the first month still have diastolic pressures above 100 mm Hg are offered drug treatment at this stage, with the aim of bringing the diastolic pressure below 90 mm Hg. Those whose pressures remain above 140/90, but stay below 150/100, are given general advice, along the lines of Chapters 4, 5 and 6.

If, after six more months, people in the general advice only category still have pressures between 140/90 and 150/100, they will usually be offered a mild drug treatment to bring down their diastolic pressures below 90 mm Hg. This is the target of all drug treatment, and indeed of all management of high blood pressure. Those whose pressures continue to rise up beyond the diastolic level of 100 during this six month period are transferred to the permanent drug treatment group straightaway.

At this point it must be emphasized, yet again, that the decision to start drug therapy is an *addition* to the change in life-style which you should have undertaken in those first months of medical supervision. I suspect that many people would rather stick to their old habits, and take drugs because it seems the easy way out, but it is the wrong one, as it will not reduce your risk of heart disease. It is also important to understand that once you do start taking drugs for hypertension, you are committed to life-long treatment and blood pressure checks. Your best chance of reducing your drug dosage, and possibly of stopping the drugs altogether, is to change your life-style. After all, your real aim is not simply to adjust your blood pressure, but to avoid the consequences of a constantly raised pressure on the circulation in your heart, brain and kidneys described in Chapter 3. The only way to be sure to do that is to co-operate in everything your doctor advises, and that includes the life-style advice, as well as the drugs.

Once the decision to use drugs has been made, the final question the doctor will ask himself is: *what drug or combination of drugs shall I prescribe?*

There is a vast array of drugs to treat high blood pressure, so that what follows may at first seem difficult. The drugs in current use are divided into groups with different actions, and within each group are listed the generic, or official, names, followed by the proprietary, or trade, name (in brackets). Examples are the beta blocker atenolol (Tenormin) and the calcium antagonist nifedipine (Adalat). It is customary for the official name to be spelled with a small first letter, and its trade name with a capital first letter.

The pattern of drug treatment

In general, doctors employ what is known as the 'stepped care' approach to prescribing for high blood pressure. This means that first you are given a relatively mildly acting drug to lower your pressure gently. After a month or so, your blood pressure will be re-assessed. If it is now normal, you remain on this first drug, in the same dose, for a few more months, until your doctor judges it is time to try to reduce it. You may be lucky, and one day be able to stop taking the drug completely, or you may have to continue for months, years, or even the rest of your life.

Whatever happens – even if you no longer need drugs – you will have to resign yourself to regular checks of your pressure for the foreseeable future. It may only be once a year for someone settled to a normal pressure on no drugs, but it is usually once a month for the others.

Second step treatment

Most people settle well on their first drug, and can continue on that single prescription, with a diastolic pressure in the 80s or 90s. For some, however, the small initial dose of the first drug does not lower the pressure enough to bring it into the normal range. They will either be offered a higher dose of the same drug, or the addition of another drug of a different type. This is the second 'step' in their treatment.

Third step treatment

Again, most who proceed to the second step settle well, and need no further treatment. This leaves a small group of people whose blood pressures have not responded satisfactorily, or who have experienced side-effects from their first treatments. They proceed to the third 'step' of taking a third group of drugs, or combination of drugs. As there are several groups of drugs to choose from, there is always some way of reaching reasonable blood pressure levels.

Once 'stabilized', either at the first, second, or third

step, you will probably remain on those drugs, at those doses, for months – but your repeated blood pressure measurements will be the guide to any change. Never ask for or accept a repeat prescription for them from your doctor's receptionist without having your pressure taken, because it may have risen or fallen, without you noticing any difference in the way you feel. It takes only a minute or two to measure blood pressure, and this is certainly not wasted time.

Your doctor bases his choice of drug for you on two guidelines.

1 He uses drugs with which he is familiar, in terms of his knowledge of their effects, their doses, and their side-effects. No doctor, however experienced, can be totally familiar with every drug for high blood pressure, so your doctor will concentrate on a few that he hopes will cover any eventuality in his experience of hypertension. So don't be surprised if a colleague, also under treatment for hypertension, but from another doctor, has different tablets from yourself.

2 Treatment depends on your type of high blood pressure. Although most fall into the 'essential' classification (see Chapter 1), some of the rarer forms of hypertension – especially those associated with phaeochromocytoma and adrenal gland disorders (again, see Chapter 1) – need specific drugs outside the usual stepped care routine. Don't be at all distressed if this is your case: these treatments are usually just as effective as the stepped care approach.

Types of drugs

Antihypertensive drugs can be divided into several groups:

Diuretics – drugs that deplete the volume of fluid in the body, thereby lowering the load that the heart has to pump around the body.

Sympathetic system blockers – drugs that reduce the nervous stimulation to the heart muscle, thereby slowing the rate at which it beats and reducing the force of the beat.

Vasodilators – drugs that open up the small blood vessels in the arms and legs, lessening the work to be done by the heart.

ACE inhibitors – drugs that block the release of angiotensin-2 into the blood (see Chapter 1). Angiotensin-2 is the body's mechanism for keeping the blood pressure normal: some people with high pressure have either too much angiotensin-2 or are too sensitive to its normal level.

Calcium antagonists – Drugs that reduce the amount of calcium inside the heart muscles and the muscles around blood vessels, thereby reducing the tension within them. This reduces the force of the heart beat and opens up the circulation in the arms and legs, lowering resistance to the blood flow within them.

Diuretics

A powerful 'natural' diuretic is to cut down on salt intake (see Chapter 4). That is the first step of all for many people with high blood pressure. If that does not bring it down to satisfactory levels, then the first drug of choice is either a diuretic or a sympathetic blocking agent, usually a 'beta-blocker'.

Diuretics increase the flow of urine and cause the kidneys to excrete sodium (salt is sodium chloride) from the body. The result is a drop in the body's water and salt levels, which in turn leads to the fall in blood pressure described in Chapter 1.

Because diuretics make you pass more urine than normal, you will be advised to take them only once a day, in the mornings. That makes sure that the effect is over before night, so that you can sleep undisturbed by a filling bladder. If you forget your morning diuretic, and take the dose after midday, expect to be wakened from your sleep.

There are three types of diuretic:

- thiazides, which are relatively mild
- 'loop' diuretics, so called because of the structure in the kidney on which they act
- 'potassium sparers'.

A problem of the first two is that, besides causing the body to lose water and sodium, their prolonged use also lowers the body's supplies of potassium. Potassium is important, among other things, in controlling the efficiency of muscle contractions, including those of the heart, so that it is common to give potassium supplements with thiazide and loop diuretics.

As their names suggest, the potassium sparers do not cause potassium excretion, so supplements are unnecessary. However, they may not be as effective as the others in lowering high blood pressure, and their effects tend to wear off, so they are rarely used alone, as a first choice. They are usually combined with either another type of diuretic, or with a drug from another group.

The table below lists the main diuretics used in hypertension:

Diuretics used in hypertension

Thiazides

bendrofluazide	(Aprinox, Berkozide, Centyl, Neo-Naclex, Urizide)
chlorothiazide	(Hygroton, Saluric)
chlorthalidone	(Hygroton)
clopamide	(Brinaldix)
clorexolone	(Nefrolan)
cyclopenthiazide	(Navidrex)
hydrochlorthiazide	(Direma, Esidrex, HydroSaluric)

hydroflumethiazide	(Hydrenox)
indapamide	(Natrilix)
mefruside	(Baycaron)
methychlothiazide	(Enduron)
metolazone	(Metenix)
polythiazide	(Nephril)
quinethazone	(Aquamox)
xipamide	(Diurexan)

Loop Diuretics

bumetanide	(Burinex)
ethacrinic acid	(Edecrin)
frusemide	(Diumide, Dryptal, Frumil, Frusetic, Lasix)

Potassium Sparing Diuretics

amiloride	(Midamor, Moduretic)
spironolactone	(Aldactone, Diatensec, Spiretic, Spiroctan)
triamterene	(Dyazide, Dytac, Dytide, Frusene)

Side-effects of diuretics are usually minor. The thiazides may cause an occasional rash, and have very rarely been reported to cause temporary falls in the numbers of white cells in the blood, but these recover if the drugs are stopped. People with diabetes, gout or liver problems are given diuretics with caution, as all three forms of diuretic can aggravate all these conditions.

Another occasional side-effect of diuretics is impotence, so if you find that your sex life is being affected, while taking them, do not hesitate to tell your doctor. A change to another drug may well help. Do not blame your impotence on your blood pressure, or on your age – even if you have reached mid-life or older.

Drugs acting on the sympathetic system

The general name applied to these drugs has nothing to do with the usual idea of 'sympathy'. It refers to the sympathetic nervous system, the network of nerves controlling the dynamics of the circulation, from the centre of the brain through the nerves to the heart, and to the muscles round the small blood vessels in the limbs and organs. Sympathetic blockers cut across the impulses in this system, making it less active. They are subdivided mainly according to where they act on the system:

- Centrally acting drugs, affecting the control centre in the brain. These are not strictly 'blockers', but act in a complex way on the nerves deep in the brain.

- Peripherally acting drugs affecting the nerves running from the spinal cord.

- 'Beta' and 'alpha' blockers, acting at the heart and blood vessels.

Today, the beta-blockers are the drugs of choice among the 'sympathetic' acting class. The others are largely obsolete because of unacceptable side effects, or because the dose has to be raised steeply as the body becomes accustomed to them, and the blood pressure starts to rise again.

The alpha blockers, indoramin (Baratol), doxazosin (Cardura), prazosin (Hypovase) and terazosin (Hytrin) are usually reserved as third line treatment to be added when the first two choices have not fully worked. The other alpha blockers, phenoxybenzamine and phentolamine, are used almost exclusively for the very rare condition of phaeochromocytoma, described in Chapter 1.

For a very few people, the 'central' and 'peripheral' drug may be prescribed only because the patient has taken it for years, still feels comfortable on it, and the blood pressure remains under control. However, most will now have been switched to the newer, more effective and less troublesome beta-blockers. The central and peripheral agents still on prescription (many have been removed in recent years) are in the table below, for the sake of completeness:

'Sympathetic' agents

Central

clonidine	(Catapres)
methyldopa	(Aldomet, Dopamet, Hydromet)
reserpine	(Decaserpyl, Serpasil)

Peripheral

bethanidine	(Esbatal)
debrisoquine	(Declinax)
guanethidine	(Ismelin)

Alpha blockers

doxazosin	(Cardura)
indoramin	(Baratol)
prazosin	(Hypovase)
terazosin	(Hytrin)
phenoxybenzamine	(Dibenyline)
phentolamine	(Rogitine)

Beta blockers

acebutolol	(Sectral)
atenolol	(Tenormin)
betaxolol	(Kerlone)
bisoprolol	(Emcor, Monocor)
labetalol	(Trandate) – also an alpha blocker
metoprolol	(Betaloc, Lopresor)
nadolol	(Corgard)

oxprenolol	(Trasicor)
penbutolol	(Lasipressin) – also contains Lasix
pindolol	(Visken)
propranolol	(Inderal, Berkolol)
sotalol	(Beta-Cardone, Sotacor)
timolol	(Betim, Blocadren)

Combinations of beta blockers and diuretics abound. They include: Co-Betaloc, Inderetic, Lopresoretic, Moducren, Prestim, Sotazide, Tenoretic, Trasidrex, and Viscaldix. Doctors prefer to reserve them for patients who find it difficult to take a host of different drugs. (Some older people may be taking drugs not only for their hypertension, but also for heart problems, or arthritis, or other unconnected long-term disorders – and the combined preparations are then very useful.)

Side-effects of the sympathetic blockers Any drugs with such a range of powerful effects on the nervous system and brain inevitably have some undesirable effects.

● The 'central' group tend to make you woolly-headed, dry-mouthed, depressed, have tummy upsets, retain fluid, have fainting spells, and if you stop clonidine suddenly, your blood pressure can shoot up again, sometimes dangerously.

● The 'peripheral' group's main problem is that they seldom completely control the blood pressure without causing unacceptable fainting attacks when you move from a lying or sitting position to stand up. Also, they can cause quite embarrassing facial flushes.

● The alpha blockers may affect co-ordination, making it difficult to drive or operate machinery.

● Beta blocker problems usually arise in people with conditions in addition to their high blood pressure. For instance, if you have bad circulation in your limbs, beta blockers may make this worse. An exception to this is labetalol, which has the extra property of opening up the small vessels in the legs.

Probably the most serious side-effect of beta blockers, and the one least often reported by the person taking them, is impotence. As with impotence related to diuretics, people are often embarrassed to talk about their sex lives, even to their doctors. If you are affected, don't suffer in silence – and unnecessarily. There are other treatments which avoid this effect.

Asthmatics are usually advised to avoid beta blockers, as they can bring on an attack, although acebutolol, atenolol and metoprolol are less likely than the others to make you wheeze. Diabetics, too, must take beta blockers with care, and may have to alter their dose of insulin to cope with lower than normal blood sugar levels. In very large doses, some beta blockers have been reported to cause vivid dreams and even hallucinations.

It would be perfectly understandable if, as you are about to start on your first course of drugs for hypertension, this list of possible side-effects puts you off taking them. Don't let that happen. These side-effects are listed, not to frighten you, but to make you aware that they may occur, and to show that if you *are* among the few who experience them, you can be switched to another treatment. If you know what may happen on the drugs, you are better able to cope, because you will know that the way you feel is not because your high blood pressure is getting worse, and you don't have to go on suffering such reactions.

The vasodilators
These are usually kept as third step drugs, because they are more effective given with others than alone. But they are sometimes the first choice in hospitals, given by injection, to bring down quickly dangerously high pressures in people admitted as emergencies.

The vasodilators used outside hospital include the alpha blockers prazosin, terazosin, doxazosin and indoramin, and two others, hydralazine (Apresoline) and minoxidil (Loniten). People taking them must be watched carefully, partly because they usually have moderate to severe high blood pressure, and partly because they can have dramatic side effects.

The first dose of the alpha blockers, for example, may cause a very sudden, steep drop in pressure, causing a faint from which it can be difficult to rouse the patient. They are therefore started at very low doses, in hospital. Fainting attacks, drowsiness and weakness are common to all these drugs.

Minoxidil is never given without a diuretic, such as a thiazide, as it causes the kidneys to retain fluid. It may also cause unwanted facial hair growth in women, a side effect that has been exploited in a minoxidil-containing ointment (Regaine) for early baldness or hair loss in both sexes.

ACE blockers
The first ACE blocker, captopril (Capoten), was initially restricted to use in severe high blood pressure. Now that it has been prescribed widely for several years, it is recommended for mild to moderate hypertension, and is given in severe hypertension when other drugs have failed or are inappropriate. It has a curious, rare, side effect that it does not seem to share with the ACE inhibitors that followed it – a loss of the ability to taste food. Not surprisingly, many people who developed this side effect stopped taking it.

Newer ACE inhibitors include quinapril (Accupro), lisinopril (Carace, Zestril), perindopril (Coversyl), enalapril (Innovace), and ramipril (Tritace). None seem to offer any great advantage over any other, or over captopril. Their side effects, generally, include rashes, cough, headaches, and nausea, as well as rare allergic reactions.

They are reserved for persons failing to respond to, or who cannot take, other treatments.

Calcium antagonists
The calcium antagonists now in general use for high blood pressure include verapamil (Cordilox, Securon, Univer), nifedipine (Adalat, Coracten), nicardipine (Cardene), amlodipine (Istin), and israpidine (Prescal). Verapamil differs from the others in that it is not usually prescribed along with beta-blockers, as the combination has caused very low blood pressures. Nifedipine, on the other hand, has been combined with a beta-blocker in two preparations, Tenif and Beta-Adalat.

Side effects of calcium antagonists include flushing and headaches, which will usually disappear after a day or two if they are continued, and should not return.

Choosing the treatment
The ever-widening range of drugs for hypertension presented the medical profession with a practical problem. How were they to decide what was best for the majority of patients?

No one physician could possibly provide the answer from his own experience: for a definitive statistical analysis of the results of all the different treatments, over many years, the data from many thousands of cases had to be included.

This is precisely what was undertaken by the British Hypertension Society in 1987. This group of seven doctors, including five professors from British universities, studied the results from worldwide trials in around 60,000 patients with high blood pressure. They came to six very definite conclusions. Doctors, they said, should:

● Treat patients under 80 years old with diastolic pressures over 100 mm Hg for three to four months (drug treatment in older persons has to depend on individual cases).

● Observe patients with diastolic pressures of 95 to 99mm Hg every three to six months.

● Use either diuretics or beta-blockers as first line treatment.

● Use other agents if these are contraindicated, ineffective, or poorly tolerated.

● Warn all patients against smoking and heavy alcohol intake.

● Advise weight reduction in obese patients.

The aim of treatment, the authors added, was to bring the diastolic pressure down to between 85 and 90mm Hg.

Writing in the *British Medical Journal* in November 1990, Professor J. D. Swales of Leicester University, Chairman of the Working Party, supported and explained these conclusions. The choice of diuretics or beta-blockers as first line treatment was taken, he wrote, because they 'have been shown beyond dispute to reduce the risk of stroke in hypertensive patients'. He added that 'the incidence of myocardial infarction (heart attack) was reduced by antihypertensive treatment'.

He continued: 'We have no evidence from trials of the effect of the newer classes of drugs – that is the ACE inhibitors, calcium antagonists and alpha blockers – on either strokes or heart attacks.'

Professor Swales touched on another aspect of treatment that is of growing importance – the cost of treatment to society as a whole. 'A year's course of bendrofluazide costs £2–£4: for calcium antagonists or ACE inhibitors the figure is £100–£200. Between 20% and 30% of the adult population are candidates for lifelong antihypertensive treatment, and the new contractual arrangements [in the British NHS for general practitioners] will inevitably encourage doctors to identify more of these patients.'

He stressed that newer drugs may or may not be better

than the betablockers or diuretics, but that it would be 'an expensive speculation that multiplies the cost of treating hypertension more than 50–fold, particularly when a substantial proportion of the adult population is affected'.

The balance in the choice between diuretics and beta-blockers, Professor Swales felt, has tended to move in favour of the beta-blockers, despite their greater cost. Treating patients with beta-blockers during or after heart attacks, he wrote, undoubtedly reduces the risk of death and further attacks, and many high blood pressure patients have established heart disease. An extra support for this view comes from the British Medical Research Council Trial published in 1987, in which the patients given a beta-blocker had fewer heart attacks than those given either placebo or diuretics.

ACE inhibitors, calcium channel blockers and alpha blockers, according to Professor Swales, have a 'substantial role' when betablockers or diuretics fail or are poorly tolerated.

He finds it difficult to believe how these conclusions can change in the next decade, in the absence of harder clinical evidence. As no new trials comparing the newer with the older drugs are now under way, I can only agree with him.

Even if the position were to change in favour of the newer drugs, Professor Swales pointed out, changing to them could only be at the expense of 'considerable impact on the care of patients with other conditions'. In these times of cash-constrained Health Services, not only in Britain, but in many other countries, budgets for drugs have assumed much greater importance than in the past. Prescribers now have to justify their prescriptions in terms of costs and subsequent benefit, and the equation falls clearly on the side of the diuretics and beta-blockers. Even in societies in which drug costs are paid for by the patient, this is one area where paying more, for newer drugs, is unlikely to reap any benefit.

Special cases – age, gender and other risks

Past advice on treating high blood pressure has differentiated patients by age, gender and other risk factors. Older patients, it was said, for example, should not be treated so vigorously, or perhaps not at all, for fear that the drop in pressure might provoke a thrombosis.

This has been proved wrong. People benefited from pressure reduction right up to the age of 80 years, so that there is no justification for withholding treatment on the grounds of age. In fact, those aged from 60 to 80 probably benefit most, in that they appear to have extra protection from strokes. However, they tolerate the drugs less well and tend not to comply as well with their dose instructions, so they need more doctor/nurse care, and probably a less drastic initial reduction in their pressures.

A common past piece of advice was that younger women with high blood pressure were better protected against strokes and heart attacks than older women or men of any age. It was therefore reasoned that they needed less treatment under the age of 50. This has turned out not to be true. When the trials were analyzed, there was just as big a reduction in strokes for women, at all ages, as for men. So all high blood pressure should be treated, regardless of gender.

Among the other risks which increased the rate of stroke and heart attack in patients with high blood pressure, such as diabetes, high cholesterol levels, a strong family history of heart disease and smoking, the trials showed that one stood out far above the others. Smoking.

The importance of stopping smoking cannot be over-emphasized. The risks of smoking outweigh the benefits of antihypertensive treatment – unless smokers stop, their risks of early death from heart attack and stroke continue as high as before, despite successful reduction in their blood pressure.

The salt saga – the final word?

We have already discussed the part played by salt in producing high blood pressure (see above, pp. 47–51). In 1990, the International Hypertension Society came to the conclusion that a general reduction in salt intake could not be proved to have any substantial effect on the number of persons having strokes or heart attacks.

This advice changed sharply on 6 April 1991, with the publication in the *British Medical Journal* of three reports of studies of the blood pressure and salt intake of 47,000 people in 24 different communities throughout the world. The authors, Professor N. J. Wald, Dr M. R. Law, and their statistician, Mr C. D. Frost, all of St Bartholomew's Hospital, London, found that in the 33 trials they studied in which people restricted their salt intake for 5 weeks or more, there were always substantial falls in blood pressure. People aged from 50 to 59 years who reduced their salt intake by only 3 grams a day lowered their high systolic pressures by as much as 7mm, and their diastolic pressures by more than 3 mm. On this basis, a similar reduction in salt intake by the whole Western world would reduce the incidence of strokes by 26% and of heart attacks by 15%.

Reducing salt by this amount can be achieved simply by not adding salt to food in cooking, and not adding salt at the table. The St Bart's team claimed that simply persuading people to do this would be more effective than using blood pressure–lowering drugs alone to prevent stroke and heart disease. They added that reducing the amount of salt added to processed foods would lower blood pressure by twice as much, and prevent some 70,000 deaths a year in Britain, as well as much disability!

Their data is very persuasive. It has to be concluded that we should all, whether we have high blood pressure or not, review our salt intake. Most of us take too much.

8

Symptoms You Should Not Ignore

As has been repeated several times in previous chapters, high blood pressure is not a disorder that causes sudden emergencies, or an abundance of unpleasant symptoms. There are problems, however, which could apply to anyone being treated for high blood pressure. They relate to the high blood pressure itself, to its complications and to its treatment.

In itself mild or moderate high blood pressure rarely causes any symptoms. This is one reason why too many people, given drugs to control it, soon stop taking them, and drift away from their doctor's supervision. The fact that they often feel worse on treatment than off it, that the whole management of their condition means considerable changes in their life styles, from eating less and more wisely to taking more exercise and stopping smoking, discourages them. They either are unwilling or unable to follow instructions – and they give up.

Try not to be like that. By neglecting your high blood pressure, you may be quietly allowing your heart and circulation to deteriorate – and the next symptom could be a heart attack or stroke. Do take to heart what your doctor says, and follow his or her advice to the letter. Remember, although the doctor can give you good advice – *you* have to follow it to give yourself the best chance of a long and healthy normal life.

There are symptoms that no hypertension sufferer should ignore, because they relate to the organs most at risk from uncontrolled hypertension:

● Dizzy spells, clumsiness, loss of balance, morning headaches, deteriorating vision, all combine to suggest problems with the circulation in the brain.

● Weakness of the limbs, especially one-sided, or of one side of the face, or of a hand, or slurred speech may be warning signs of stroke, which treated quickly, can be averted.

● Increasing breathlessness on exercise, with pains in the chest, running into the jaw, arm, back or upper tummy, suggest the beginnings of angina.

● Becoming generally breathless, so that you find it easier not to lie flat, with boggy swelling in the feet and ankles, could be the other trouble associated with high blood pressure: heart failure.

● Having to rise every night to pass urine, and passing more urine, more frequently, during the day, may be the first sign of kidney problems.

All these symptoms are quite different from the side-effects of the drugs you may be asked to take (see Chapter 7). Recognize them as possible warning signals, and do talk them over with your doctor. There may be simple explanations for the symptoms so that you need nothing more than reassurance. Even if you *are* developing trouble, it is usually because your blood pressure has not been completely controlled. When this is recognized early and treated appropriately, all the complications of the disease can be reversed, and the symptoms cleared. If you neglect them, however, they will worsen.

Sadly, the main reason for such deterioration in health can all too often be the patient's own fault. More than in any other illness, people with high blood pressure either forget to take their treatment, or deliberately stop taking it. They either feel so well that they don't see why they should carry on with the treatment, or the side-effects bother them too much. It is in your own best interests to realize that in all probability your blood pressure will never be 'cured', and will need lifelong management if it is to be contained.

If you do *not* take your medicines regularly, as advised, your blood pressure will not be fully under control. Damage may continue unrecognized, while you believe you are perfectly well. There is really no excuse for not taking the modern drugs – most need only be taken once, or at most twice, a day, and if you do experience side-effects, there are alternative drugs your doctor can try.

If you do tend to forget your pills, despite your best intentions, link taking them with some routine act you perform at roughly the same time every day, such as brushing your teeth or setting your bedside alarm. You might consider buying one of the modern watches with a built-in alarm, to remind you of your pill time, wherever you happen to be.

As an insurance, wherever you go, keep with you, in your wallet or handbag, a note saying that you have high blood pressure and giving details of the drug you are taking. It is not a pleasant thought, but you may one day be involved in an accident, and need urgent treatment. If you have to be given drugs, your casualty surgeon and anaesthetist should know what you have taken already that day, so that they know which drugs they must avoid, and which they may use safely.

Finally, a word of reassurance. High blood pressure is not a disease in itself. It is only an indication that, if it is not controlled, you are at higher than usual risk of certain medical problems, such as a stroke and heart attacks. The aim of treatment – and of the advice given in this book – is to reduce those risks to the low levels enjoyed by people with normal blood pressure. Once you and your doctor have worked together to control your hypertension – with your changed life-style, and perhaps with drugs – you have every prospect of a long and healthy life.

Appendix

Measuring Blood Pressure with the 'Sphygmo'

There is little mystery about the sphygmomanometer, or 'sphygmo', as it is usually called. It consists of a cloth cuff enclosing an air-proof bag, inflated via a tube from a rubber bulb inflator, to which is connected a device which measures pressure – this may be a reservoir of mercury leading to a vertical glass tube, or a pressure gauge similar to that on a barometer.

The cuff is wrapped around the patient's upper arm, and the bag inside the cuff is inflated by rhythmically squeezing the bulb. The pressure inside the cuff rapidly rides to above the pressure in the artery in the upper arm, preventing the flow of blood through the artery. Anyone listening with a stethoscope over the site of the artery in the crook of the elbow when the cuff pressure is above the systolic pressure, will hear nothing.

If the listener then releases the valve at the bulb, the pressure in the cuff falls slowly, until suddenly the sound of the pulse can be heard beating in the artery. The point at which the sound breaks through – and it is usually very easy to define – is the systolic pressure, that is, the pressure exerted on the circulation by the heart. At this stage, the cuff pressure is still higher than the diastolic pressure – the sound the listener hears is that of the sides of the artery slapping together as the blood passed through and the artery virtually empties with each beat.

As the cuff pressure is lowered still more, the beats heard via the stethoscope becomes muffled, then disappear altogether. The pressure at which the sounds disappear is the diastolic pressure – now the blood is flowing continuously in the artery, and the walls no longer meet to produce a sound.

The whole exercise takes only a few seconds in experienced hands, but do remember not to wear clothing with a tight sleeve when you attend for your check-up. This not only wastes the time when you try to roll the sleeve up, but it can itself constrict the arm, leading to a falsely low, and even possibly dangerously misleading, reading on the sphygmomanometer.

The simplicity of the process is such that anyone can be trained to measure the blood pressure accurately enough to be a guide to treatment. Self-measurement of blood pressure has been taken up by tens of thousands of people in the United States and in Europe, but to a much lesser extent in the United Kingdom. The reason for the reticence of the British to follow their transatlantic cousins is not clear, but it may be partly due to the fact that we can see our doctors, for no fee, and have our blood pressures checked at the intervals suitable to our needs.

There is some truth, too, in the attitude of many British doctors, who believe that overemphasis on the height of your blood pressure can make you a 'blood pressure neurotic', obsessed by every small rise and fall. Once you are stabilized, there seems little point in measuring your blood pressure more than once a month.

In the first few months, however, knowing how to take your own blood pressure may be a great help to your doctor, while he or she is deciding which treatment to prescribe. A diary of measurements, taken at first several times a day, then later several times a week, could show how well you respond to different treatments. It could also show you how your blood pressure responds favourably to changes in your daily routine – and in so doing perhaps strengthen your resolve to stick closely to your new life-style.

If the idea of taking your own pressure interests you, discuss the possibility with your doctor. He or she can advise you on whether it will be worthwhile for you, and if so, how to do it, how often, and which type of machine to buy. The mercury machines are easier to maintain, and probably stay accurate for longer than the cheaper aneroid devices, the gauge accuracy of which needs to be checked every six months. Whichever you do buy, it is very important that you follow closely the manufacturer's instructions on maintenance.

The size of the cuff, too, is important. If you are overweight, or have a large, thick upper arm, choose a wide, long, cuff which fits round it comfortably. If the cuff is too narrow, it may give a falsely high reading. A normal-sized cuff will suit thin adult arm, but special cuffs are needed for small children – take the child with you to ensure that you buy a cuff of the right size.

Also, the stethoscope should be light and fit closely and comfortably into your ears. And you should be able to hear clearly through it! Sphygmomanometers can be bought with stethoscopes attached, specially designed to allow self-examination. Sphygmomanometers cost around £50, and stethoscopes about £15–£30. There is no need to buy more expensive instruments, as these offer no advantages for you in accuracy or reliability.

Index